MIASMATIC DIAGNOSIS

PRACTICAL TIPS WITH CLINICAL COMPARISONS

(Including Summary of Miasmatic Indications from Head to Foot with Psychic
& Paediatric Manifestations and Miasm-Medicine Chart)

by

DR. SUBRATA KUMAR BANERJEA

Gold Medalist

B.H.M.S. (Honours in Nine Subjects of Calcutta University).
Fellow : Akademie Homoopathischer Deutscher Zentralverein (Germany).
Director : Bengal Allen Medical Institute.
Principal : Allen College of Homceopathy, Essex, England.

B. JAIN PUBLISHERS (P) LTD.

An ISO 9001 : 2000 Certified Company
USA — EUROPE — INDIA

Reprint Edition: 2004, 2005, 2006, 2007

MIASMATIC DIAGNOSIS

Revised Edition: 2003

© Copyright with the author

Published by

Kuldeep Jain

for

B. Jain Publishers (P) Ltd.

1921, Chuna Mandi, St. 10th Paharganj,
New Delhi-110 055
Ph: 2358 0800, 2358 1100, 2358 1300, 2358 3100
Fax: 011-2358 0471
Website: www.bjainbooks.com, Email: bjain@vsnl.com

PRINTED IN INDIA
by
J. J. Offset Printers

BOOK CODE ISBN 978-81-319-0073-4

BOOKS BY SAME AUTHOR

☞ Synoptic Memorizer of Materia Medica

☞ B.H.M.S. Solved Papers Pharmacy Including Viva-voce & Practical Parts

☞ Essential Guide to Materia Medica

☞ B.H.M.S. Solved Papers on Anatomy Including Dissection & Viva-Voce

☞ Materia Medica made easy Abis canadensis-Digitalis

☞ Brain Tumor Cured by Homoeopathy

☞ Schematic Comparison of Remedy

☞ Clinical & Comparative Materia Medica

☞ Repertorial Analysis and Evaluation

About the Author

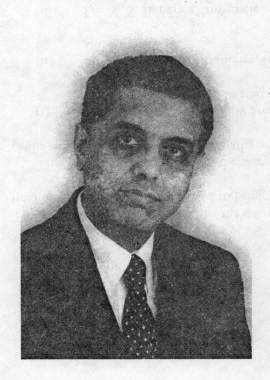

Dr. Subrata Kumar Banerjea was born in Calcutta, India in 1957, the fourth generation of a distinguished and widely respected homoeopathic family. He graduated in Homoeopathy from the University of Calcutta with a record number of honours passes in nine medical subjects and with five gold medals to his name, setting himself on a path to become an internationally acclaimed homoeopathic clinician, lecturer and author. He is now acknowledged to be the world's leading authority on miasmatic prescribing.

Dr. Banerjea is an Honoured Fellow of several academies; Director and Principal Lecturer of the Bengal Allen Medical Institute, Calcutta; Principal and Chief Lecturer of Materia Medica and Clinical Therapeutics at the Allen College of Homoeopathy, Essex, England. When he is not lecturing, he divides his time between his clinical practices in the UK and in India where he also acts as Clinical Consultant in various rural and slum clinics.

Despite this hectic international scheduling, Dr. Banerjea together with his brother Joy and his partner Janet Robinson, plays an active role in the Kamala Banerjee Fund, a charity which distributes milk to the poor children of Calcutta.

Students of Dr. Banerjea will testify to the remarkable knowledge and enthusiasm which he generously imparts to all who share his passion for this most rational of healing arts. His dedication to the truth of homoeopathy is regarded as inspiring and unsurpassed.

Dedication

This book is humbly dedicated to the sacred memory of my mother, Late Dr. (Mrs.) Kamala Banerjee, whose un-stinting co-operation and unending patience in every regard to bring me up and her constant inspiration was the "golden key" of all my achievements and laurels.

This book also commemorates the sacred memory of my three generations of homoeopathic ancestors, who have dedicated their lives for the cause and development of Homoeopathy and to them Homoeopathy was "wealth and honour".

(i)   Dr. Kalipada Banerjee, (my great grandfather), Founder Proprietor, C. Ringer & Company, Calcutta (Homoeopathic Chemist & Druggist of a century old tradition).

(ii)   Dr. Kishori Mohan Banerjee, (my grandfather), Founder of Bengal Allen Homoeopathic Medical College & Hospital, Calcutta and

(iii)   Dr. N. K. Banerjee, (my uncle), Principal, Bengal Allen Homoeopathic Medical College, Calcutta; President, Homoeopathic State Faculty, West Bengal and Indian Homoeopathic Association; Author of : A Treatise on Homoeopathic Pharmacy; Practice of Medicine, etc.

Essex, England.
Dated :10th April, 2002.
Hahnemann's Birthday.

Dr. Subrata Kumar Banerjea

Preface

I was born and brought up in a homoeopathic family and in an environment of homoeopathic philosophy and am proud to say that homoeopathy is in my blood. I am a fourth generation homoeopath, my great-grandfather Dr. Kalipada Banerjee was born in a town near Calcutta (India) in 1844 and was a practising homoeopath for 38 years. His son, my grandfather, Dr. Kishori Mohan Banerjee, was born in 1886 and followed in his father's footsteps qualifying as a homoeopath in Calcutta, which by this time had acquired a reputation as the 'Mecca of homoeopathy'. My grandfather however, had a great desire to broaden his knowledge and travelled to America where he learned the art of miasmatic prescribing directly from the great Dr. John Henry Allen. After returning to his native country, Dr. Kishori Mohan Banerjee founded The Bengal Allen Homoeopathic Medical College and Hospital in 1924 naming it after his much loved and respected tutor, Dr. Allen. Sadly, he died at the young age of 55 but his legacy lived on through his son, my uncle, Dr. Naba Kumar Banerjee, by whose inspiration my own love of homoeopathy was discovered and nurtured. Although my father Dr. R.K. Banerjee is a pathologist, he has always rendered support in my studies of this great art and science of homoeopathy, as has my aunt, Dr. Kamala Banerjee, whose love and affection was key to many of my earlier academic laurels. My family have always held true to Hahnemannian-Kentian principles and since my grandfather's time incorporated miasmatic diagnosis into their plans of treatment. It is this approach, which I believe, was intrinsic to their success as homoeopathic physicians and I offer you this book not only in their memories but also for the future of homoeopathy.

The inclusion of miasm in a homoeopathic prescription is becoming more and more important in this modern world of suppression. Hahnemann with his infinite wisdom recognised some two hundred years ago the prominence of one-sided diseases with a scarcity of proper characteristic symptoms, and the increasing usage of modern drugs has intensified this to a degree that such cases are becoming increasingly common today. There can only be one approach if a complete cure is sought and this is to systematically remove each layer of suppression and miasmatic dyscrasia before proceeding to nip the underlying cause of disease in the bud.

This book is designed for homoeopathic practitioners and students alike and for this reason I am assuming a degree of knowledge as befits both. However, I feel it is worthwhile at the outset to define the homoeopathic context of the word miasm as an invisible, inimical, dynamic principle, an inherited weakness, a stigma or vacuum in the constitution and to share with you the analogy of the peeling away of petals from the lotus flower, a representation of the removal of each different layer of suppression or disease and their corresponding dyscrasia which I use in my lectures to demonstrate the curative art of miasmatic prescribing.

With proper application, miasmatic prescribing can uproot the underlying cause of disease and nip the bud of increased susceptibility to future diseases, so it is not only curative but also preventative, something for which our patients will surely thank us in the long run. There are no shortcuts to complete and permanent cure and it is up to us and our patients to play our parts in striving towards successful treatment in as many cases as possible. It is by the incorporation of miasmatic prescribing into our treatments that this can become possible.

There are two main sections to this book as detailed below :

Part I — Miasmatic Diagnostic Classifications: Starting with the mental symptoms, this is a head to foot schematic classification of the four miasms, including my tips for rapid miasmatic diagnosis.

Part II — Miasmatic Weightage of Medicines: A comprehensive guide to the weight, value or gradation of the medicines and listings of the leading anti-miasmatics.

I have worked for many years in completing this book and in last twenty-two years or so, have lectured on miasms all over the world wherever homoeopathy is known. It is always a pleasure to lecture on Miasm as I can share my great love and passion for this subject. This venture however would not have possible without the constant support, care and co-operation, love and affection of my partner Janet and I am deeply touched and indebted to her.

I would also like to sincerely acknowledge the help given by Debasish Mukherjee for his technical support in typing the manuscript and M/S Jain Publishers for their help with the printing and publishing this book.

I welcome any constructive suggestion towards the improvement of future editions. All the information mentioned herein has some verifications and it is with this foreknowledge and my own experience that I have been successfully incorporating miasmatic prescribing into my practices for many years. I entreat you to publish the failure of Miasmatic incorporation in prescribing, if any and if ever, to the world!

It is my hope that you will both learn from and enjoy this book and that the benefits of prescribing miasmatically will be experienced by both yourselves and your patients.

Subrata Kumar Banerjea
Essex, England.
10th April, 2002
(Hahnemann's birthday).

MIASM

Dr. Banerjea's Definition

I define miasm as an invisible, inimical, dynamic principle, which permeates into the system of a living creature, creating a groove or stigma in the constitution, which can only be eradicated by a suitable anti-miasmatic treatment. If effective anti-miasmatic treatment does not take place then the miasm will persist throughout the life of the person and will be transmitted to the next generation.

MIASM

Dr. Banerjea's Ten Principles

I.   Miasm is a dynamic energy, which cannot be seen.

II.   Every living creature on earth, bacteria, virus etc., has its own miasm.

III.   Miasm is hostile to the life preserving energy (inimical to the vital force) of any living creature.

IV.   It is dynamic, as it affects the dynamic plane and thereby dynamically deranges the life preserving energy of any living creature.

V.   The basic pre-condition of a miasmatic infection is susceptibility.

VI.   When a person or any living creature is susceptible (characterised by hypo-immunity = psora) the inimical, invisible dynamic principle of miasm gets the chance to permeate into the body (as the immunity is low and thereby the person is susceptible to receive such infection), this is known as miasmatic infection.

VII.   After entering in the body, it tends to join the fundamental miasms already existing in the body.

VIII. Then it takes the upper hand; as the miasmatic force from outside plus the miasmatic force already dormant in the body conjoin together and dynamically affect the vital force (life preserving energy) thereby dynamic derangement of the vital force occurs.

IX.   So the miasmatic force dynamically deranges the vital force, and that results in disease. There is always a battle going on inside the body between the vital force and the miasmatic force; in health the vital force wins and in disease, the miasmatic force wins.

X.   The miasmatic force creates a stigma or vacuum in the constitution, which can only be eradicated by suitable anti-miasmatic medicine, otherwise it is transmitted to the next generation. Miasmatic dissection and incorporation of the same in each case will help (a) to open up a case, where there is a scarcity of symptoms due to various physical, emotional or iatrogenic suppressions, by the centrifugal action of deep acting anti-miasmatic medicines. Also of importance is the value of selecting an anti-miasmatic medicine, which covers the nature and character of the individual in absence of any recognisable totality. Thus, the anti-miasmatic medicine covers the essence of the person and opens up the case; (b) to be more confident in prescribing by including the surface miasm in the consideration of the totality, as miasm, the dyscrasia of the person, constitutes a major part of the totality; (c) to evaluate the necessity of change of the plan of treatment or change of the remedy; as few symptoms have disappeared after the first remedy, yet the miasmatic totality indicates the preponderance of the same miasm in the surface which was originally covered by the initial remedy, therefore it foretells that we can stay with the previous remedy; (d) to evaluate the homoeopathic prognosis of the case, as removal of layers of suppression manifest as clarity of symptoms and can be accompanied by a quantum jump in the sense of well being; (e) to fulfil Hahnemann's three injunctions of cure: rapid, gentle and permanent; and (f) anti-miasmatic medicines help to clear up the suppressions (in relation to the past); clear up the presenting symptoms from its root or origin (in relation to the present); and clear up the susceptibility to get infection and thereby strengthens the constitution (in relation to the prophylactic aspect or future).

Why Should We Know Miasm?

A thorough dissection and incorporation of miasm in each case will help a homoeopathic prescriber in the following ways:

(i)   A deep acting anti-miasmatic medicine by virtue of its centrifugal action will open up such cases (brings to the surface the suppressed symptoms) where the totality of symptoms cannot be framed due to a scarcity of symptoms (i.e. one-sided cases), and those cases with conjoint or contaminated pictures due to various physical, emotional or iatrogenic suppressions.

(ii)   Also of importance is the value of selecting an anti-miasmatic medicine, which covers the psychic essence, nature and character of the individual in absence of any recognisable totality. For example, a patient presents with insomnia with no distinguishing modalities or other characters to complete the symptom. By ascertaining that person's psychic essence or character (for instance, suspicious, jealous and exploiting in nature, representing sycosis) we can prescribe an anti-miasmatic medicine to cover the insomnia and open up the case. Thus, the anti-miasmatic medicine covering the essence of the person is capable of surfacing the suppressed symptoms and the totality can then easily be framed.

(iii) To be more confident in prescribing by including the surface miasm of the case in the consideration of the totality; as miasm, the dyscrasia of the person, constitutes a major part of that totality. Miasm and the symptoms are nothing but the two sides of the coin, and one cannot be considered whilst ignoring the other. In fact, the totality of symptoms cannot be said to be total until and unless the selected remedy covers the miasm.

(iv) To evaluate the necessity of a change in the plan of treatment or a change of remedy; when few symptoms have disappeared after the first remedy has been administered, yet the miasmatic totality shows the preponderance of the same miasm on the surface as that which was originally covered by the initial remedy. It indicates that the prescriber can stay with that initial remedy, as can be seen from the following example: a patient came with the presenting symptom of facial wart, for which Causticum was prescribed. As this medicine covers the miasm (here in this case, sycosis) as well as the symptom, the wart has fallen off; and the next suppressed layer, perhaps a profuse yellowish leucorrhoea (which was previously suppressed by cauterisation) comes to the surface. This symptom too is a sycotic manifestation, and is also covered by Causticum, then that remedy will totally eradicate the problem. So knowledge of miasm guides us to stay with the remedy and to allow its full and complete action.

(v) To evaluate the homoeopathic prognosis of the case, as removal of layers of suppression are manifested as clarity of symptoms and also reflected by a quantum jump in the sense of well-being. Deep acting anti-miasmatic medicines by virtue of their centrifugal action will remove the layers of suppression which can be evidenced as follows:

a) A quantum jump in the sense of well being.
b) Improved energy.
c) Increased appetite.
d) Better quality of sleep.
e) Harmony and tranquillity of temperament.
f) Stability (in obese people) or weight gain in under weight subjects.
g) Clarity of the existing or presenting symptoms or even lighter symptoms.
h) Suppressed symptoms (even of years ago) reappear on the surface and are permanently eradicated. This reappearance can be in a very transient form, which may not even be visible to the naked eye.

(vi) To fulfil Hahnemann's three injunctions of cure: rapid, gentle and permanent.

(vii) Anti-miasmatic medicines help to clear up the suppressions (in relation to the past); clear up the presenting symptoms from their root or origin (in relation to the present); and clear up the susceptibility to get infection and thereby strengthening the constitution (in relation to the prophylactic aspect or future).

Contents

PART — I : MIASMATIC DIAGNOSIS : MIASMATIC DIAGNOSTIC CLASSIFICATIONS 1

1. Miasmatic Diagnosis: Comparison of the Mental Symptoms 1
2. Miasmatic Diagnosis: Comparison of Characteristics and Nature 12
3. Miasmatic Diagnosis: Comparison of Vertigo Symptoms 20
4. Miasmatic Diagnosis: Comparison of Head & Scalp Symptoms 22
5. Miasmatic Diagnosis: Comparison of the Eye Symptoms 30
6. Miasmatic Diagnosis: Comparison of the Ear Symptoms 33
7. Miasmatic Diagnosis: Comparison of Nasal Symptoms 36
8. Miasmatic Diagnosis: Comparison of the Oral Symptoms 40
9. Miasmatic Diagnosis: Comparison of the Facial Symptoms 43
10. Miasmatic Diagnosis: Comparison of the Respiratory Symptoms 46
11. Miasmatic Diagnosis: Comparison of the Cardiac Symptoms 52
12. Miasmatic Diagnosis: Comparison of the Stomach Symptoms 56
13. Miasmatic Diagnosis: Comparison of the Abdominal Symptoms 62
14. Miasmatic Diagnosis: Comparison of the Rectal Symptoms 65
15. Miasmatic Diagnosis: Comparison of the Urinary Symptoms 70
16. Miasmatic Diagnosis: Comparison of the Sexual Symptoms 74
17. Miasmatic Diagnosis: Comparison of the Dermatological Symptoms 82
18. Miasmatic Diagnosis: Comparison of the Nail Symptoms 89
19. Miasmatic Diagnosis: Comparison of the Extremity Symptoms 90
20. Miasmatic Diagnosis: Comparison of Sleep Symptoms 96
21. Miasmatic Diagnosis: Comparison of Modality Symptoms 98
22. Miasmatic Diagnosis: Comparison of Characteristics: A Synopsis 100

PART — II : MIASMATIC DIAGNOSIS : MIASMATIC WEIGHTAGE OF MEDICINES 118

PART — III : MIASMATIC DIAGNOSIS: LEADING ANTI-MIASMATIC MEDICINES 126

PART — I
MIASMATIC DIAGNOSIS :
MIASMATIC DIAGNOSTIC CLASSIFICATIONS

MIASMATIC DIAGNOSIS:
COMPARISON OF THE MENTAL SYMPTOMS

	Key Word	Inconsistent Psoric Mind	Avaricious Sycotic Mind	Destructive Syphilitic Mind	Dissatisfied Tubercular Mind
1.	Introduction	Diversion, perversion and reprobation of the mind to commit evil are the primary manifestations of psora. For this reason the psoric mind is always outwardly manifesting and there can be no deep mental concentration, meditation or sacred thoughts.

The 'hypo' psoric state is manifested in the mental sphere as hypo-reasoning, i.e. inconsistent, impractical thoughts and hypo-confidence that results in anxieties and all varieties of fears.

Anxiety, inconsistent thoughts, apprehension (especially of impending misfortune) and alertness are therefore the basic criteria of the psoric mind. | The Sycotic taint develops the worst forms of debasement because of its basic suspicion and jealousy. It has the tendency to harm others, even animals (especially mentally in the form of mental torture).

Sycotic mental symptoms are either 'hyper', or characterised by incoordination. Examples are: hyper-workaholics, hyper-greedy (avaricious) & hyper-rageous types and those showing an incoordination in behavior like jealousy and/or suspicion. A tendency to exploit may also be present. | The syphilitic miasm has a destructive mentality, which perverts, deforms and vitiates the senses of judgement, the memory and the sharpness of the intellect. The patient can neither realise the symptoms nor can he explain them to the physician. In any such case where the patient cannot explain his symptoms, describe their character, or iterate his desires and aversions, the syphilitic stigmata will be present.

Syphilitic mental symptoms are characterised by destruction and even love for one's own life is destroyed leading to suicidal tendencies. There are impulses towards destruction and violence. | Dissatisfaction and lack of tolerance are the innate dyscrasias of the tubercular stigmata.

Lack of tolerance leads to anger and irritability, which in time results in depression.
The dissatisfied state of the mind makes him changeable both mentally and physically and manifests in the following manners:
Persons can never be satisfied in a certain job or place, or with a certain subject or situation. Children desire this or that, especially toys, but when offered, they out rightly reject them and demand something new.
Students frequently change their subjects — perhaps studying |

				science for some time and then changing to arts.
				People continuously desire new jewellery and clothes. They are always finding new passions and cravings, and never find peace or satisfaction in any one object.
				Persons crave and have perversions (this perversion is afforded by the syphilitic component of the tubercular miasm) for the things that will harm them, wanting for example, foods which aggravate their condition.
				Dissatisfaction resulting in changeability is the innate dyscrasia of tubercular miasm.
2. Thoughts & Flow of Words	The psoric attitude towards religion is deceitful and the patient appears as a feigning philosopher due to his inability to concentrate. There may be a passionate craving or indulgence to obtain unnecessary objects and a tendency to build castles in the air! Thoughts and words overflow in the mind, and accordingly, words are multiplied.	This miasm produces the worst forms of cruelty and in this respect is similar to the syphilitic miasm. However, with sycosis there is also cunning deceit and the worst form of manias of all the stigmatas. Men and women who commit suicide are mainly syphilo-sycotic. Sycosis is the most mischievous of all the miasms. Sycosis cannot find the right	Destruction, perversion, dissolution or degeneration are the most significant characteristics of syphilis. Syphilitics are generally close mouthed and may answer in monosyllables. They lack ideas, expressions and thoughts due to destruction of the intellectual capabilities. Suicidal planning and thoughts are syphilo-sycotic but when suicides are committed without	A lack of concentration, and thoughtlessness regarding appearance is representative of the tubercular miasm.

Key Word	Inconsistent Psoric Mind	Avaricious Sycotic Mind	Destructive Syphilitic Mind	Dissatisfied Tubercular Mind
		words and if he does, he is not sure whether they are right. He has doubts about his spelling and experiences difficulty in narrating his symptoms. All the fascists and exploiters of the world are the product of syphilis.	any planning and in a manner devoid of intelligence then the syphilitic miasm is evident on the surface.	
3. Awareness	Psoric patients are mentally alert, and are quick and active in their motions. They will work like 'Trojans' for a short time, but become easily fatigued both mentally and physically and a profound prostration follows. The fatigue is accompanied by the desire to lie down and extreme fatigue restrains them from performing their duties. Heat of the whole body follows mental impressions or exertions. The patient is sensitive to odours and atmospheric changes and is easily disturbed mentally.	Sycotic patients are always suspicious, a taint which can manifest in a variety of ways. They may be suspicious of their surroundings and of other people. They are even suspicious of their own work and do not trust themselves to the extent that they must go back and repeat what they have previously done or said, and wonder if they have said just what they mean. This suspicion when turned upon others, leads to the worst forms of jealousy. They may be jealous of both their family and friends. In the case of injury, the patient themselves will examine the site of the lesion very carefully and frequently and keep changing physicians.	Mentally dull, heavy, stupid and especially stubborn. Idiocy, ignorance and obstinacy lead to melancholia and gloominess. Mentally slow to react, and if reading for example, they can read only a few lines, which they must read again to fully comprehend. What they read they cannot retain — a kind of mental paralysis.	Tubercular children manifest their traits in the extreme. They may be either slow or dull and experience difficulties in comprehension or they may be very bright, intelligent and alert.

Key Word	Inconsistent Psoric Mind	Avaricious Sycotic Mind	Destructive Syphilitic Mind	Dissatisfied Tubercular Mind
4. Anxiety	Psoric patients are anxious to the point of worry and fear. Anxiety on awakening in the morning which may at times compel them to move about.	Anxiety from changes in the weather and from humidity typifies the sycotic patient.	In syphilis, anxiety occurs at night.	The mental changeability and dissatisfaction of the tubercular patient ends in a depressed state of mind which is striking in the fact that even in this depressed state there is a total absence of disappointment, hopelessness, anxiety or apprehension. Tubercular patients do not worry about anything, even when suffering from the most severe ailments
5. Cruelty	Real cruelty is not typical of the psoric mentality, but there can exist deceitful behaviour with a tendency to make others appear foolish.	Cruelty, mostly in the form of mental tortures, lack of affection, rudeness and vexation are all present in sycosis. Anger from trifles may lead to physical assault. The sycotic patient tries to hurt others emotionally. Sycosis is also present in such instances as where a family suffers because the mother cannot accept her daughter-in-law, and in businesses where employer/employee relations are regularly strained.	Syphilitics are the cold-blooded murderers, the committed criminals and iconoclasts. Physical destruction, bodily assaults, killings and physical tortures are the product of syphilis.	Some cruelty may exist in the tubercular miasm due either to the patient's innate dissatisfaction or from the tubercular combination of psora and syphilis. Tubercular children may exhibit some features of cruelty through physical and mental torture of their friends and/or siblings.

Key Word	Inconsistent Psoric Mind	Avaricious Sycotic Mind	Destructive Syphilitic Mind	Dissatisfied Tubercular Mind
6. Fears	Almost all the fears have a psoric base and these fears manifest as anxiety. Psoric patients are easily frightened, often by trivial things, which lead to trembling and perspiration followed by great weakness. In children there may be fear of darkness, fear of strangers, fear of many fictitious things and fear of animals. They are timid about going to school and their fears become so intrinsically interwoven into their lives that very soon they wear themselves out and become thoroughly exhausted. As a result, mental growth becomes stunted and this in turn affects their physical growth. Adult fears include a fear of death on becoming ill, fear of incurable diseases and fear that they will be unable to accomplish what they attempt. There also occurs sudden anxiety in the region of the heart, particularly when stomach conditions are present.	Sycotic fears are manifested outwardly. There is a fear of making mistakes, so the sycotic patient repeatedly checks what they have done.	The syphilitic patient fears people and conversation due to their own dullness and idiocy. Their gloominess is manifested through anxiety and apprehension and fear is manifested through anguish.	The tubercular miasm is generally fearless although there is an innate fear of dogs.

Key Word	Inconsistent Psoric Mind	Avaricious Sycotic Mind	Destructive Syphilitic Mind	Dissatisfied Tubercular Mind
7. Memory	As psora is 'hypo' in its manifestation so it shows as a weakness of memory.	There is absentmindedness and abstraction of thought in sycosis. A general loss of memory, losing the thread of the conversation, forgetting words and sentences and the previous line just read are characteristic of sycotic incoordination. They often forget recent events but can remember the events of distant past. There may also be momentary loss of thought and slowness of speech.	Syphilitic patients lack a sense of duty and responsibility and often fail to perform family duties due to impaired memory. There is also a lack of self-confidence. Love of one's own life is a natural instinct of man, but the syphilitic patient, due to impaired memory, a lack of self confidence and self-awareness believes there is no way left other than to commit suicide. Syphilis shows forgetfulness and a total destruction of memory. Arithmetical calculation is difficult.	Memory problems, especially in children, result from a lack of tolerance and manifest as a difficulty in comprehension and retaining facts. They are often labelled as problem children, due to their lack of patience and tolerance and their inability or slowness to comprehend. They find it difficult to try again and there is a continued dissatisfaction. On the other hand, tubercular children can also be very bright and show great keenness of intellect.
8. Social Interaction	There is an aversion to people and company, especially unknown people. However, the psoric patient also dreads being alone. Roams in deserted places.	Sycotics are the extroverts but in all cases of deprivation and rudeness sycosis is present. It is the most mischievous of all the miasms for its jealousy, exploiting nature and tendency to mentally torture others. Despite their extrovert nature, sycotic patients show a lack of self-confidence in social interactions.	Syphilitic patients are introvert and have a great desire to escape from both themselves and from others people. Their desire for solitude and aversion to company can lead to suicidal tendencies. Syphilitics lack self-confidence and do not trust others. Due to dullness of intellect, loses the thread of conversation and lacks perception.	Tubercular patients sometimes appear as morose and sullen. They do not like receiving advice from others, especially with regards to their health.

Key Word	Inconsistent Psoric Mind	Avaricious Sycotic Mind	Destructive Syphilitic Mind	Dissatisfied Tubercular Mind
			Syphilitics are close-mouthed and do not worry their friends with their troubles. They regard both the death of an individual and the explosion of a nuclear bomb over a town as appropriate.	
9. Restlessness	Mental restlessness to achieve unnecessary objects is one of the primary manifestations of psora.

Psoric anxiety and fears give way to mental restlessness and in turn the patient feels compelled to move about.

Psoric patients are not direct thinkers except for a very short time. Thoughts come thick and fast so that they entangle them and they cannot maintain a particular train of thought for any length of time. This mental restlessness causes them to complain they want to do something but they do not know what they want to do. Activities are both started and ended in a dramatic way.

Psoric restlessness is particularly noticeable at the new moon and in the case of | The restlessness and dissatisfaction present in this stigmata manifest in a more physical form.

Sycotic patients frequently change their posture and cannot keep quiet or still. | Mental restlessness (a psoric component must also be present) drives the patient out of bed and induces symptoms of suicide.

Restlessness can be great but is devoid of any realisation or understanding. | Dissatisfaction is the innate dyscrasia of this miasm, which results in changeableness and a restlessness, manifested both mentally and physically.

Tubercular patients move home frequently and move from place to place or from town to town, travelling even when strength does not permit. They change occupation, doctors, even their furniture and the arrangements of their rooms, always with a constant desire to do something differently.

This constant changeableness results in mental fatigue, which in turn manifests as an apathetic, indifferent state of mind. The patient may, without notice, up and leave to live as a vagrant due to their dissatisfaction with everyday life and the policies of the world. They can be seen |

Key Word	Inconsistent Psoric Mind	Avaricious Sycotic Mind	Destructive Syphilitic Mind	Dissatisfied Tubercular Mind
	women, at the approach of the menses. A peculiar characteristic of the mental irritation is that it produces a sense of bodily heat and these patients have flushes of heat while working.			sagging down on pavement with fatigue but will jump up on seeing a dog.
10. Attitude	The psoric miasm shows a selfishness and lack of human conscience. Patients may internally be extremely selfish, but on the outside appear to be very liberal. Rich people, for example, may hide their wealth by dressing down and shrewd people may pretend to be religious and make huge charitable donations. Hide and seek is in the nature of psora. Psoric patients have a tendency to dishonesty and secretiveness; wickedness and impurity will be present.	Sycotic patients have a suspicious attitude towards their surroundings, their family and friends and even to their own work. They are jealous and as a result want to commit detriment and mental torture to other people. Sycotics are the fascists and exploiters of the world. They are possessive and selfish people with a tendency to conceal.	Syphilitics are close-mouthed, melancholic individuals who are continually depressed and constantly dwell on suicide. They are merciless in nature and have no sympathy for anything, including themselves. An urge for destruction seems to be their only emotion. The syphilitic patient lacks a sense of duty and therefore appears unconcerned about their family and relations. However, this is due to the destruction of their sense of realisation, intellect and memory meaning that they cannot realise their duties.	The careless, apathetic, indifferent attitude of the tubercular patient is a reflection of their desire for self-destruction and a suicidal impulse is manifested through this general indifference. They are unconcerned with, or indifferent towards the seriousness of sufferings, and if the suffering is their own, they are always hopeful of recovery. The unrestrained, uncontrollable passions of life, such as masturbation, artificial loss of semen and perverted cravings for sex are adopted by this patient, leading to great debility and the way to an early grave. These unrestrained passions are also characterised by indifference to every thing.

Key Word	Inconsistent Psoric Mind	Avaricious Sycotic Mind	Destructive Syphilitic Mind	Dissatisfied Tubercular Mind
11. Intellect	Thoughts seem to vanish whilst reading and writing. The psoric patient seems unable to control their thoughts, which sometimes seem to disappear altogether.	Sycosis shows an abstraction of memory and an incoordination in thoughts and perceptions.	In the syphilitic miasm, destruction of the intellectual capabilities results in total forgetfulness and a loss of sense of realisation.	With the manifestation of tubercular polarities comes a state of opposites where patients may be either intellectually sharp or totally dull.
12. Behaviour	Indolent patients with an aversion to working and bathing are psoric. They lack discipline, are untidy in appearance and averse to keeping things clean. Time goes either too fast or too slow.	The sycotic patient is always thinking about their own ailments and has difficulty in remaining under the treatment of one physician alone. However, there is also a tendency to suppress their ailments or symptoms. Their behaviour reflects their basic suspicious, jealous, quarrelsome, mischievous, selfish, rude, mean-minded and concealing nature.	The close-mouthed syphilitics are merciless, destructive and violent in their behaviour. Children's minds remain immature and they have a fear of strangers.	Tubercular patients are apt to behave in an indifferent, dissatisfied, changeable, careless or fearless manner. They do not like advice in regards to their health or diet due to their innate dissatisfaction and desire for change.
13. Temperament	Psora shows a change of temperament without any apparent cause. Young people particularly become hysterical especially after acute weakening diseases. Fits of anger alternate with a tearful mood but with this anger there is seldom any desire to harm others. The fits are usually accompanied with trembling followed by great prostration (+++) after which they may	In sycosis, the slightest change of temperature reflects as changes in the mind. Anger is aggravated by changes of weather, particularly from thunderstorms and the sycotic miasm is aptly termed as 'the living barometer'.	Syphilis has fixed ideas, which are not eradicated by any amount of talk or explanations. Perversion and destruction of the intellectual functions result in obstinacy as a marked result of fixed idea and in fixed moods. Depression is always present but syphilitic patients keep their troubles to themselves and sulk	The tubercular patient is extremely irritable and fearful and even becomes frightened and disgusted when looking at their own image. This further fuels their innate desire for change. Patients may be extremely outrageous, foolhardy and impatient which results in quarrelsomeness (syco-tubercular).

	remain sick for quite some time. Psoric patients suffer from a depression of spirits in which they burst out crying to relieve the condition. When in this state, everyone knows of their troubles, as they are unaccustomed to silent grief. However, some psoric patients become so depressed that they are unable to speak. There is a changeableness in psora although the tubercular stigma is usually behind when changeability is manifested to such a large extent. The psoric patient is a chronic complainer, never satisfied with the conditions in their lives.		over them. They remain immersed in melancholia and depression, which leads to an anxious state in which they prefer to be in solitude. Syphilitics are the cold-blooded iconoclasts.	Mental symptoms, especially anger, are worse after sleep and the patient may wake with a feeling of dissatisfaction clearly visible on their face.
14. Criminality	Feigning, deceitful philosopher types are the product of psora.	Sycosis in combination with psora is the basis of most criminal insanities.	A combination of syphilis and sycosis results in sullen, smouldering patients, threatening to break out into dangerous behaviour at any time.	The fearless tubercular patient is unconcerned and indifferent but willing to take risks and undertake ventures.

Key Word	Inconsistent Psoric Mind	Avaricious Sycotic Mind	Destructive Syphilitic Mind	Dissatisfied Tubercular Mind
15. Manias	Psora, with all its anxieties and fears is very likely to develop some manias.	In sycosis there are many manias, which are all, characterised by underlying suspicion. E.g. the patient may check the room again and again to see that no one is hiding behind the cupboard or they may check the lock repeatedly. They may also repeat the same word or sentence, thinking that others cannot understand them, even to the extent of returning to an acquaintance after they have just parted to ensure that they were correctly understood.	Syphilis is characterised by violent and destructive rages and manias.	Even the manias of the tubercular miasm are changeable and patients may change such things as ornaments, clothes, curtains, occupations, household furniture and the arrangement and decor of the room.
16. Modalities	The psoric patient is ameliorated by natural discharges and from the appearance of suppressed skin conditions.	Sycotic mental conditions are aggravated by changes in the weather and humidity and much ameliorated when warts or fibrous growths appear or when old ulcers or sores break open. There is a marked amelioration of all symptoms by the return of suppressed gonorrhoeal manifestations.	In syphilis, the mental symptoms are aggravated at night and ameliorated by unnatural discharges.	All tubercular mental symptoms are aggravated by thunderstorms and ameliorated in open air.

MIASMATIC DIAGNOSIS:
COMPARISON OF CHARACTERISTICS AND NATURE

Key Word	Psora Sensitising Miasm	Sycosis Miasm of Incoordination	Syphilis Degenerating Miasm	Tubercular Responsive, Reactive Miasm
1. General Manifestations	i) Psora develops itch.	i) Sycosis develops catarrhal discharges.	i) The syphilitic miasm has virulent open ulcers.	i) The tubercular miasm has haemorrhages.
	ii) Unhealthy skin with burning and itching represents psora.	ii) Oily skin with thickly oozing and copious perspiration, represents sycosis.	ii) Ulcerated skin with pus and blood represents syphilis.	ii) Oily skin with coldness represents the tubercular miasm.
	iii) All 'hypos' are mainly psoric.	iii) 'Hypers' are sycotic.	iii) 'Dyses' are syphilitic.	iii) Allergies are tubercular.
	iv) Hypoplasia is psoric.	iv) Hyperplasia is sycotic.	iv) Dysplasia is syphilitic.	iv) Alternation of 'hypo' and dysplasia is tubercular.
	v) Atrophy, ataxia, anaemia and anoxaemia are psoric.	v) Hypertrophy is sycotic.	v) Dystrophy is syphilitic.	v) Dystrophy with haemorrhage is tubercular.
	vi) Hypotension is psoric.	vi) Hypertension is sycotic.	vi) Irregular, arrhythmic pulse is syphilitic.	vi) Intermittent pulse is tubercular.
	vii) Lack, scanty, less and absence denote psora.	vii) Exaggeration or excess denotes sycosis.	vii) Destruction and degeneration denote syphilis.	vii) Alternation and periodicity is tubercular.
	viii) Weakness is psoric.	viii) Restlessness (especially physical) is sycotic.	viii) Destructiveness is syphilitic.	viii) Changeableness is tubercular.
	ix) An inhibitory tendency is psoric.	ix) An expressive tendency is sycotic.	ix) Melancholic, depressive and suicidal tendencies are syphilitic.	ix) A dissatisfied tendency is tubercular.

Key Word	Psora Sensitising Miasm	Sycosis Miasm of Incoordination	Syphilis Degenerating Miasm	Tubercular Responsive, Reactive Miasm
	x) Dryness of membranes denotes psora.	x) Augmented secretion denotes sycosis.	x) Ulceration denotes syphilis.	x) Haemorrhages and allergies denote the tubercular miasm.
	xi) Psora does not assimilate well.	xi) Sycotics are over-nourished.	xi) Syphilitics have disorganised digestion.	xi) Tubercular types crave the things which make them sick.
	xii) The secretions of psora are serous.	xii) Sycotic secretions are purulent.	xii) Syphilitic secretions are sticky, acrid and putrid.	xii) Tubercular secretions are haemorrhagic.
2. General Nature of the Miasm	Hyper-sensitivity (basically psora is 'hypo' in expression which leads to low immunity resulting in hyper-susceptibility. This manifests as an exalted sensitivity to external allergens and environment). Itching, irritation and burning lead towards congestion and inflammation with only functional changes. The capacity to produce hypersensitivity or in other words the sensitising property of psora is the basic nature. By dint of this property it makes the organism susceptible to all sorts of environmental conditions and diseases, as well as to allergens.	Sycosis produces incoordination everywhere, resulting in over-production, growth and infiltration in the form of warts, condylomata, tumours and fibrous tissues etc.	Syphilis produces destructive disorder, which manifests as perversion, suppuration, ulceration and fissures.	The tubercular miasm produces changing symptomatology and confusing vague symptoms (e.g. dyspepsia, weakness, wasting and fever). Manifestations are variable, shifting in location, alternating in state and contradictory.

Key Word	Psora Sensitising Miasm	Sycosis Miasm of Incoordination	Syphilis Degenerating Miasm	Tubercular Responsive, Reactive Miasm
3. Key Words and Expressions	Hypo-immunity. Anxiety. Apprehension. Alertness. Fears. Irritation—mental and physical. Sensitivity.	'Hyper' — mental and physical. Hypertrophy; growths; incoordinations.	Destruction — physical and mental. Degeneration. Necrosis and ulceration. Putridity and acridity. 'Dyses'. Irregular; arrhythmia.	Dissatisfaction. Alternation; changeability; migratory. Periodic. Recurrence. Allergic. Vague manifestations. Craves the things which make them sick.
4. Diathesis	i) Eruptive diathesis.	i) Rheumatic and gouty. ii) Lithic and uric acid. iii) Proliferative diathesis.	i) Suppurative or ulcerative diathesis.	i) Scrofulous diathesis. ii) Haemorrhagic diathesis. iii) Allergic diathesis.
5. Organs and Tissues Affected	Ectodermal tissues. Nervous system, endocrine system, blood vessels, liver and skin.	Entodermal and soft tissues. Attacks internal organs, pelvis and sexual organs, and the blood (producing anaemia).	Mesodermal tissues. Soft tissues and bones; glandular tissues particularly the lymphatics.	Glandular tissue. Patient is poor in bone, flesh and blood.
6. Nature of Diseases	i) Deficiency disorders.	i) Deposition and/or proliferation of cells/tissues.	i) Destructive, degenerative disorders, deformities, fragility.	i) Depletion. ii) Drainage and wastage. iii) Alternating disorders.
7. Pace of Action	i) Hyperactive. ii) Dramatic development of symptoms.	i) Extremely slow, insidious. ii) Silent or even surreptitious in its manifestations.	i) Usually midway in pace, i.e. moderate. Though sometimes rapid and/or sometimes can be insidious. ii) Generally more overt in its manifestations.	i) Depends according to preponderance of psoric or syphilitic miasm.

Key Word	Psora Sensitising Miasm	Sycosis Miasm of Incoordination	Syphilis Degenerating Miasm	Tubercular Responsive, Reactive Miasm
8. Constitution	Carbonitrogenoid (excess of carbon and nitrogen).	Hydrogenoid (excess of water).	Oxygenoid (excess of oxygen).	Changeable constitution with alternation and periodicity.
9. Psychic Manifestations				
a) The person	The sterile philosopher who has lots of ideas but cannot materialise them. Theoretical persons with no sense of practicality at all. Dishonesty, secretiveness, wickedness and impurity play a large part in the psoric nature.	Deceitful, sullen, cunning persons are sycotic. They are very practical, have a tendency to exploit others and care only for their own benefit and pleasures.	Syphilitic persons seem to have one emotion only–the urge for destruction. They lack any sense of realisation, duty and understanding. Syphilitics are the committed criminals and cold-blooded murderers. They suffer from a vitiated mentality, which impairs their sense of judgement.	The tubercular person is always dissatisfied and changeable. They display both a lack of tolerance and of perseverance.
b) The nature of the miasm and the person	Psora is the sensitising miasm in that, hyperactivity and hypersensitivity of the mind and body result from increased susceptibility due to hypo-immunity.	Sycosis is the miasm of 'hyper' and incoordinations. These 'hyper' states result in abnormal behaviours and mental incoordinations such as extreme jealousy, loquacity and selfishness.	The destructive syphilitic patient has no love for their own life and either destroys themselves or kills others. They can be both suicidal and cold-blooded murderers. Syphilitics lack mercy and sympathy and may be called iconoclasts.	The changeable tubercular miasm results in dissatisfied patients who are changeable both mentally and physically.
c) Work	Quickly fatigued with a desire to lie down is characteristic of the psoric miasm. Patients may also be indolent.	Sycotics are hyper-workaholics.	Syphilitic patients show no interest in work due to their lack of realisation and understanding.	The changeable, impatient tubercular types are unable to concentrate on work.

Key Word	Psora Sensitising Miasm	Sycosis Miasm of Incoordination	Syphilis Degenerating Miasm	Tubercular Responsive, Reactive Miasm
d) Behaviour	Psora is fearful, anxious, alert and apprehensive. Nervous persons are psoric.	Sycosis is quarrelsome, jealous, selfish and cunning with a tendency to harm (emotionally) others and to harm animals. The sycotic patient may be ostentatious and fatuous, suspicious of his own work and surroundings. Mischievousness, meanness, and selfishness summarise the essence of sycosis.	Syphilis is cruel, destructive and perverted and may do harm to themselves or others.	Fearlessness and an absolute lack of anxiety are denominating features of the tubercular miasm. Patients are careless, unconcerned and indifferent about the seriousness of their sufferings and always hopeful of recovery.
e) Memory	Weakness of memory indicates psora.	Absentmindedness is sycotic. Patients lose the thread of the conversation. They are apt to forget the recent events but can remember the events of the past.	Forgetfulness is syphilitic. There is a kind of mental paralysis, the patient may read but cannot retain the information. The mind is slow.	Changeableness of thought and perception is tubercular.
f) Death	Fear of death is psoric. There is also anticipation and anxiety regarding death.	Suicidal patients are mainly syphilo-sycotic. The sycotic patient will plan their death but are unlikely to commit suicide as their attachment to life and will to live is usually too strong.	The syphilitic patient dwells on suicide, has suicidal thoughts and dreams and experiences the urge to commit suicide. Love for their own life is destroyed. When syphilis is coupled with sycosis it becomes the basis of most suicides and criminal inanities, and a preponderance of syphilis results in sullen, smouldering persons likely to break out into dangerous manifestations.	Dissatisfaction with life, changeableness and a vagabond mentality can lead to suicidal impulses. The tubercular instinct for self-destruction is characterised by carelessness.
g) Selfishness & Deprivation	Psora's selfish impulses lead them to deprive others (a trait which is also strongly present in	Sycosis is present in all varieties of deprivation and rudeness. In a factory for	The syphilitic lack of realisation results in patients who are unlikely to deprive others for	Irritable and outrageous behaviour with a lack of tolerance can be reflected as the

Key Word	Psora Sensitising Miasm	Sycosis Miasm of Incoordination	Syphilis Degenerating Miasm	Tubercular Responsive, Reactive Miasm
	sycosis). Deprivation may also manifest in the sense of presenting a false or pseudo-image of themselves. They donate (though not voluntarily), large sums of money to charity, hoping to benefit in some way from their 'generosity'.	example, where labour unrest is common, the sycotic manager tries to deprive the workers out of a concern for his own benefit. A sycotic person will always act in a most selfish way to deprive others.	their own benefit. However, a criminal, for example will not realise the impact that his time in prison will have on his family and is therefore selfish only in the sense of being focussed in one particular direction. The syphilitic patient with their destructive impulses, tends to forget or ignore other responsibilities.	selfish nature of the tubercular miasm.
h) Fear	All varieties of fears are classed under psora and manifest as anxiety, alertness and apprehension of impending misfortune. Mental restlessness is one of the expressions of psoric fear.	As a result of incoordination of thoughts, sycotics manifest some fears. A millionaire for example can develop a constant fear of poverty, which is expressed as selfishness, suspicion and physical restlessness.	Syphilitic fears are not properly manifested due to a lack of realisation and expression. The only possible outward feature one might expect from a syphilitic person is of anguish.	Fearlessness is characteristic of the tubercular miasm and is expressed by the patient as a complete indifference regarding their health e.g. even at the height of fever they will say, "I am fine and don't need the doctor!" There is one fear only and that is of dogs and sometimes other animals.
i) Expression	Psora is full of ideas and philosophical expression. They pile up books and switch from one to another reading only superficially. Psoric patients rarely go into any topic in depth, and although various ideas crowd their minds there is no practicality. This constant flow of ideas is a result of mental restlessness.	Jealousy and suspicion are very evident in sycotic expression, as are the tendencies to suppress and conceal. This innate suspicion means that sycotic patients do not trust anything and repeatedly check everything.	The introverted, close-mouthed syphilitic patient keeps their depression to themselves and it only becomes apparent after they have committed suicide. They have a tendency to suppress and conceal and an inability to realise and express their symptoms. Any true form of expression is lacking. Syphilitics have a desire to	With the tubercular miasm, the mental symptoms, in particular anger, are especially aggravated after sleep. A feeling of dissatisfaction is clearly manifested in their face after sleeping. Changeability, a lack of tolerance and impatience are the expressions of this miasm.

Key Word	Psora Sensitising Miasm	Sycosis Miasm of Incoordination	Syphilis Degenerating Miasm	Tubercular Responsive, Reactive Miasm
			escape from themselves as well as from others. Their own idiocy, ignorance and obstinacy lead to melancholia and gloominess. A desire for solitude can lead to depression and melancholia, resulting in suicidal impulses.	
10. **Key Words of Mental Manifestations**	i) Anxious and fearful. ii) Philosophical. iii) Irritability with anxiety. iv) Sadness. v) Nervous. vi) Thoughtful but no practical sense. vii) Lack of concentration and weakness of memory viii) Malicious = psora-syphilo-sycotic. ix) Wariness of life = psora-syphilitic. x) Illusions.	i) Suspicious and jealous. ii) Arrogant. iii) Irritability explodes into anger — the patient may bang the table and throw things and restlessness results. iv) Moaning. v) Chaos = Syco-Syphilo-Psora. vi) Thoughtfulness focussed for their own personal benefits. vii) Incoordination in concentration and absentmindedness. viii) Mischievousness = syco-syphilo-psora. ix) Tendency to exploit everything from life = sycotic. x) Delusions.	i) Destructive and melancholic. ii) Close-mouthed. iii) Irritability with cruelty. iv) Lamenting. v) Madness = Syphilo-Syco-Psora. vi) Vanishing of thoughts. vii) Total destruction of concentration; forgetfulness. Dullness is expressed as a weakness in perception. viii) Hatred = syphilo-syco-psora. ix) Loathing of life = syphilo-psora. x) Hallucinations and deliriums.	i) Changeable and fearless. ii) Indifferent. iii) Irritability with impatience. iv) Changeable mood. v) Insanity = Mixed Miasmatic with tubercular. vi) Changeability of thoughts. vii) Changeability of concentration. viii) Indifference = tubercular. ix) Unfulfilling life = tubercular. x) Vacillation of thoughts.

Key Word	Psora Sensitising Miasm	Sycosis Miasm of Incoordination	Syphilis Degenerating Miasm	Tubercular Responsive, Reactive Miasm
	xi) Sadness and depression.	xi) Irascibility, rudeness and ill-manners.	xi) Sentimental and closed-mouthed.	xi) Independent and indifferent.
	xii) Psora initiates many schemes but there are always loop-holes and plans are seldom realised. They may plan a robbery but it is unlikely to happen.	xii) Sycosis is cunning and practical and benefits at the expense of others. They can fill the loopholes and benefit from crime without appearing to be actually present.	xii) Syphilis attacks the guard and is the hired criminal. These patients fail to realise that if they are caught they will be sent to prison and that there will be no one to look after their family!	xii) The tubercular 'criminal' will commit to joining in a bank robbery but change their mind at the last moment and fail to turn up.
	xiii) The psoric memory is poor but the patient is studious and once they have learnt their subject they will remember it.	xiii) Sycotics have an active memory and are able to record everything — the journalist type.	xiii) Syphilitic patients cannot remember recent happenings but can recall past events in chronological order.	xiii) Tubercular patients are intelligent and bright but make careless mistakes.

MIASMATIC DIAGNOSIS:
COMPARISON OF VERTIGO SYMPTOMS

Key Word	Psoric Vertigo	Sycotic Vertigo	Syphilitic Vertigo	Tubercular Vertigo
1. Introduction	Psoric vertigo manifests especially from indigestion or emotional disturbances and may appear in any of the following ways: Vertigo with momentary loss of consciousness when things appear too large or small. Vertigo as if intoxicated, as if floating on air. Vertigo on reading or writing with confusion of the mind; spots or stars before the eyes or a feeling as if there is a veil before the eyes. Vertigo on riding in a boat, car or carriage, sometimes with a sensation of falling, as a result of anaemia of the brain. Vertigo on closing the eyes, disappearing on opening eyes (also sycotic).	Vertigo on closing the eyes, disappearing on opening eyes (also psoric).	Syphilitic vertigo begins at the base of the brain.	Vertigo beginning at the base of the brain can be either tubercular or syphilitic.
2. Modalities	Psoric vertigo is aggravated by movement, warmth, and as the	Sycotic vertigo is aggravated on closing the eyes and	Syphilitic vertigo aggravates at night.	Vertigo in the tubercular patient is ameliorated by rest, from

Key Word	Psoric Vertigo	Sycotic Vertigo	Syphilitic Vertigo	Tubercular Vertigo
	sun's rays increase. It is also worse from looking up suddenly and rising from a sitting or lying position and in these cases spots may appear before the eyes. Vertigo also occurs when turning over in bed and on closing the eyes. There is amelioration by rest, lying down and when the sun's rays decrease.	ameliorated on opening them.		being quiet, sleep, eating and from epistaxis.
3. Concomitants	The vertigo of psora is accompanied by temporary loss of vision, nausea and vomiting of mucus only. There is a lightness of the head when stooping. Digestive disturbances may also occur as may frequent eructation and roaring in the ears.	In sycosis, vertigo is associated with restlessness and there may also be sensations of formication (insects crawling over body) or of a living animal moving in the abdomen.	Total forgetfulness accompanies syphilitic vertigo.	In the tubercular miasm, vertigo is associated with impatience and dissatisfaction and redness (flushing) of the face.

MIASMATIC DIAGNOSIS:
COMPARISON OF HEAD & SCALP SYMPTOMS

Key Word	Psoric Head	Sycotic Head	Syphilitic Head	Tubercular Head
1. Headaches a) Introduction	Psoric headaches may result from hunger, exposure to the sun; or from suppressed eruptions.	Sycotic headaches are characterised by their appearance in the frontal or vertex areas.	In syphilis, constant headaches appear persistently on one side of the brain. They are usually basal or linear.	Tubercular headaches may occur from repelled or suppressed eruptions. They can be extremely painful, persistent and of long standing and are not easily amenable to treatment.
	One-sided headaches (also syphilitic).			In children, tubercular (and syphilitic), headaches may cause the patient to strike, knock, or pound their head with their hands or against some object.
	Long standing headaches like migraine.			Headaches appear periodically and may occur every weekend, Sunday or rest day. They can be seasonal or associated with the new or full moon and appear to be especially painful when on holiday.
	Sharp, severe paroxysmal headache.			

Key Word	Psoric Head	Sycotic Head	Syphilitic Head	Tubercular Head
b) Sensation	The psoric headache throbs and there may be a rush of blood to the head with a sensation of heat and flushing.	The sycotic headache appears with a sensation of heaviness.	The syphilitic headache is dull, heavy and persistent. It can often last for days at a time and is so severe as to be unendurable. These feelings may be accompanied by a sensation of bands around the head, a trait also shared by the tubercular miasm.	The tubercular, periodic headaches can be very severe and are sometimes accompanied with a sensation of bands around the head (also a syphilitic manifestation).
c) Modalities	The psoric headache is worse during the morning as the sun ascends and decreases in the afternoon with the sun's descent.	Sycotic headaches are aggravated after midnight, from lying down, and from physical or mental exertion. Amelioration may result from gentle motion.	Syphilitic headaches are aggravated at night, by the warmth of the bed, by rest, while attempting to sleep, riding and exertion.	Tubercular headaches are worse from motion and from preparing for examinations. There is also exacerbation from heat.
	A persistent morning headache constantly returns, usually in the frontal, temporal or tempo-parietal regions.	Headaches in the vertex or frontal regions are aggravated by lying down especially after midnight.	Syphilitic headaches occurring in the occipital or temporal regions are also aggravated at night, by rest and lying down, and during sleep.	Meeting with strangers and entertaining them or the approach of strangers causes or aggravates the tubercular headache.
	Amelioration is from rest, quiet and sleep and hot applications.	Sycotic children have headaches, which are aggravated at night and ameliorated by motion.	Headaches are better in the morning until the evening and worse again at night.	Tubercular headaches are relieved by rest, quiet, sleep, eating and by epistaxis.
	Psoric patients cannot bear much heat about the head although they like heat in general.		Cold applications, changing places, motion, and nose bleeds ameliorate. Head feels better before sleep.	

Key Word	Psoric Head	Sycotic Head	Syphilitic Head	Tubercular Head
d) Concomitants	Psoric headaches may be accompanied by bilious attacks, which come on once or twice a month.	Sycotic headaches are associated with fever, restlessness, sadness, crying, fretting and worrying.	The syphilitic headache is associated with profuse offensive sweat on the head.	Extreme weakness accompanies the tubercular headache. There may also be a deathly coldness of the hands and feet with prostration, sadness and general despondency, or a rush of blood to the head or face with hot hands and feet.
	Headaches with throbbing and redness of the face.	The patient is restless and wants to be constantly on the move, which relieves.	The syphilitic child strikes, knocks or pounds their head with their hands or against some object (a taint also present in the tubercular miasm).	With a tubercular headache comes rolling or boring of the head into the pillow and hunger either before or during the attack.
	There may be great hunger before and during a psoric headache.	Sycotic headaches are also associated with coldness of the body and prostration.		Tubercular headaches may occur with coughs, colds and coryza.
2. Migraine				
a) Location	Psoric migraines occur mostly in the frontal, vertex or temporal regions or over the whole head. They are often felt only externally (tension headaches).	Sycotic migraines occur in the frontal and vertex regions and occasionally parietal.	Syphilitic migraines are mostly occipital or temporal, although occasionally they occur in the base of brain, the internal head and the meninges.	Tubercular migraines are patchy in their distribution and may be temporal or parietal or occur in the base of the brain or the meninges.

Key Word	Psoric Head	Sycotic Head	Syphilitic Head	Tubercular Head
b) Sensation	In psora, migraines may be sharp, severe and paroxysmal. The pain may appear on one side only and is often long-standing and of a functional character.	Sycotic migraines are characterised by a dull aching, heaviness and a reeling sensation.	The syphilitic migraine is constant and persistent and often occurs at the base of the brain on one side only. The pain may be stitching, tearing, boring, digging, maddening, sharp or cutting etc.	Tubercular migraines are extremely painful and occur especially on holidays. They may migrate from the right eye to the left ear and can be caused by the approach of a stranger. There is a sensation of throbbing, or hammering, and a pressive, tightness like a band (with effusion in the meninges).
c) Modalities	The psoric migraine increases and decreases with the sun. There is aggravation in the morning, from motion, cold, hunger and anxiety. Rest, quiet, sleep, warmth (hot applications) and natural eliminations ameliorate.	The sycotic migraine shows aggravation from rest, humidity, lying down and cold. There is also a worsening of symptoms from morning to night and around midnight. Amelioration is from motion, violent exercise, warmth and abnormal discharges.	In syphilis, migraines are aggravated at night, and from evening to morning (during sleep). Hot or warm weather, the warmth of the bed, natural discharges, rest and lying down also aggravate.	In the tubercular miasm, migraines appear worse in the evening and forenoon, from cold and every change in the weather. Patients are averse to having their heads uncovered. Epistaxis, rest, quiet, sleep and eating ameliorate.
d) Concomitants	i) Mental symptoms such as fear, anxiety and apprehension. ii) Red face with throbbing of the carotids. iii) Hot flushes ending with little perspiration.	i) Urogenital symptoms. ii) Crossness, irritability and jealousy. iii) Restlessness.	i) Suicidal tendencies. ii) Imbecility. iii) Migraine may be associated with allied disturbances of the cardiovascular and nervous systems.	i) Red face with throbbing of the carotids (psora offers this symptom to the tubercular miasm). ii) Nose bleed, which relieves symptoms. iii) Migraine with cough, cold and coryza.

Key Word	Psoric Head	Sycotic Head	Syphilitic Head	Tubercular Head
	iv) Sweat on head during sleep.	iv) Vertigo, which appears on closing the eyes and disappears on opening them.	iv) Deficient blood supply.	iv) Hunger during the headache.
	v) Vertigo, aggravated by looking up suddenly, rising from a sitting position or from emotional disturbances.	v) Congestion leads to stagnation causing the arteries to become sluggish.		v) Offensive head sweats.
				vi) Extreme weakness with the migraine.
				vii) Tubercular children suffering from migraine may strike, knock or pound their heads with their hands or against some object.
				viii) Vertigo, which begins at the base of the brain.
				ix) Active congestion leading to pulsation, which shakes the whole body.

26

Key Word	Psoric Head	Sycotic Head	Syphilitic Head	Tubercular Head
3. Hair	Psoric hair is apt to be thin, dry and lustreless. It appears dead like hemp and is so dry that it must be wet before it can be combed. It can also appear matted and the ends are dry and liable to split.	Sycotic patients may suffer from a fishy odour from both their hair and their scalp.	Syphilitic hair is oily, gluey and greasy, and moist eruptions may appear in the scalp. There can often be a sour, foetid or metallic odour.	As the tubercular miasm is a combination of psora and syphilis, the hair may either be dry, rough and harsh and break and split easily (psoric preponderance) or oily and moist and stick or glue together (syphilitic preponderance). There may be a thick, yellow, heavy crust of pus or it can be moist and greasy with an offensive, musty odour.
	Alopecia can affect the psoric patient and the hair may fall out after an acute illness or fever, or after parturition.	Hair falls out, and alopecia occurs in circular, circumscribed patches. Baldness is a common feature.	In syphilis, the hair has a tendency to fall out in bunches usually on the sides of the head or the vertex.	Tubercular hair is likely to fall out after parturition.
	Hairs grey on the midline of the head, or become white or grey in spots. Greying occurs too early.	In sycosis, there is likely to be an abundance of premature grey hair or immature greyish hair.		
	Bran like dandruff with or without itching.		Dandruff with thick yellow crusts.	

Key Word	Psoric Head	Sycotic Head	Syphilitic Head	Tubercular Head
	Hair may be found over the scapula where psora is joined with sycosis.		Hair falls out from the eyebrows, eyelashes and beard, and the hairs of the beard are often in-growing. Elderly people complain that the eyelashes break and turn inward, causing much irritation to the conjunctiva.	
4. Scalp	In psora, dry eruptions, which become brown and turn into dead scales, appear on the scalp. They are often painful and burn and there is severe itching and dryness. Aggravation occurs in the open air, from the heat of the bed and during the evening. Amelioration is from scratching but burning and smarting follow.	In sycosis, vesicular types of skin eruptions appear in the scalp. There may also be warts, veruccas and tumours.	Syphilitic scalp eruptions have offensive, oozing pus and are aggravated by washing.	In the tubercular miasm, herpetic eruptions occur on scalp. They are aggravated by bathing and in the open air and there is an aversion to having the head uncovered.
5. Shape of Head	In psora the head is generally small in comparison to the rest of the body and there is a dry appearance to the hair and facial skin.	The sycotic head is large and appears over-developed. The top may appear bloated.	In syphilis, the head and ear appear long in comparison to the body. There may be delayed bony developments, open fontanelles and sutures and there is a possibility of glabellar prominence due to defective bone development.	

Key Word	Psoric Head	Sycotic Head	Syphilitic Head	Tubercular Head
6. Perspiration	Sweat on the head smells sour (++) and appears particularly during sleep, or the scalp may be dry and devoid of perspiration.	Sycotic perspiration is sour (+++) especially in children and there may be a fishy or musty odour.	Offensiveness and putridity of all the discharges are the general characteristics of syphilis and the perspiration is copious, sour (+) and foetid and may have a metallic smell.	Offensive (++) head sweats occur in the tubercular miasm and there can be a musty odour like old hay.

MIASMATIC DIAGNOSIS:
COMPARISON OF THE EYE SYMPTOMS

Key Word	Psoric Eye	Sycotic Eye	Syphilitic Eye	Tubercular Eye
1. General & Clinicals	Psoric eyes have a great intolerance of daylight and sunlight.	Corneal incoordinations and inflammations occur in sycosis.	Syphilitic eyes often have scaly red lids. They are subject to all sorts of structural changes, and also to corneal ulceration.	Tubercular eyes are characterised by granulations of the lids, haematoma in the eye and all types of inflammation characterised by haemorrhage.
	Conjunctivitis, iritis and other inflammations are of a functional nature.	Cataracts (incoordination in the lens), retinoblastoma and other papillomas and glaucoma are sycotic. Tumors, tarsal tumors and styes also occur. Ptosis is syco-syphilitic.	Retinal detachment is syphilitic.	Injury to the eyes and black eyes are tubercular.
2. Characteristics	In psora, the vision may be blurred and letters may run together whilst reading. Spots before the eyes are also characteristic of this miasm.	Cataracts can be syco-syphilitic, in that opacity of the lens is characterised by incoordination (sycosis) but degenerative changes take place when the syphilitic miasm supervenes.	Cataracts and ulceration of the cornea and lids are characteristic of syphilis.	Chronic dilatation of the pupils and sunken eyes occur in the tubercular miasm.
	The visualisation of various colours and a zigzag appearance around objects is psoric.		Paralytic weaknesses, deformities and changes in the lens and all refractory changes are syphilitic.	Changes in the lens can also be of the tubercular miasm.

Key Word	Psoric Eye	Sycotic Eye	Syphilitic Eye	Tubercular Eye
		Photophobia may occur due to condylomata, and the eyelids are often matted together in the morning.	Photophobia also occurs in syphilis and there can be an intolerance of artificial light.	Styes, photophobia and aversion to artificial lights may also be tubercular.
			Fever of ophthalmic origin.	Disturbances in the glandular structures or in the lachrymal apparatus are tubercular (and also syphilitic).
3. Sensation	In psoric eyes, there is dryness, burning and itching with a constant desire to rub the lids. There may also be a sensation of coldness or of sand-like particles in the eyes and they may be red in appearance. Conjunctival problems occur especially when there is an ardent desire to rub the eyes. Itching in the canthi is not ameliorated by rubbing.	In sycosis, eye pains manifest as dull and aching.	Syphilis shows a sensation of burning and a raw feeling in the eyes.	In the tubercular miasm there is redness in the eyes with a sensation of heat or flushing.
4. Modalities	In psora, functional disturbances are aggravated during the daytime especially in the morning and by sunshine, and are ameliorated by external warmth.	Arthritic troubles of the eye (which are a combination of sycosis and psora), and neuralgias are aggravated by changes in the weather, changes of the barometer and rain.	Syphilitic neuralgia of the eyes is aggravated by warmth and ameliorated by cold.	Tubercular neuralgias are ameliorated by warmth.

Key Word	Psoric Eye	Sycotic Eye	Syphilitic Eye	Tubercular Eye
	There is an intolerance of daylight and sunlight, and general aggravation in the morning, from the rising of the sun to its zenith. All psoric eye problems are ameliorated by heat.	Ophthalmic disorders are aggravated by changes of the season and by rain.	There is a general aggravation of eye symptoms at night and from the warmth of the bed.	Closure of the eyelids during pain ameliorates.

MIASMATIC DIAGNOSIS:
COMPARISON OF THE EAR SYMPTOMS

Key Word	Psoric Ear	Sycotic Ear	Syphilitic Ear	Tubercular Ear
1. Clinicals	In psora, otitis occurs with dryness of the meatus.	In sycotic otitis there is profuse exudation.	Syphilitic otitis is characterised by ulceration. Mastoiditis occurs with degenerative changes in the bones.	In the tubercular miasm, otitis occurs with exudation mixed with blood, cheesy or curdled.
2. Characteristics	In the psoric miasm, the meatus and canal of the ear appear dry and lustreless. Dry scales constantly come out or fall into the canal. Psoric ears may have a dirty appearance. In psora we find functional disturbances of the ear.	Sycotic ears appear swollen and thick about the pinna, and can be oedematous. Growths and anatomical incoordination are apparent about the external ear.	All structural and organic ear problems are syphilitic. Long ears. Degenerative inflammation and destruction of the ossicles of the ear is syphilitic (and can also be tubercular).	In tubercular children the ears often act as a safety valve lessening the severity of other diseases. The appearance of abscesses in the ears of such children indicates a good prognosis as for example in the case of meningitis, the abscesses help to relieve the meningeal pains. Tubercular children may appear well in the daytime but their suffering begins at night and they often awake from sleep screaming with earache. When free of ear problems, these children often suffer from throat infections.

Key Word	Psoric Ear	Sycotic Ear	Syphilitic Ear	Tubercular Ear
	Various noises in the ear are characteristic of the psoric miasm.			In tubercular patients, suppurative otitis media is a good prognosis when suffering from a severe or acute infectious disease.
				Slight exposure to the cold may result in earache leading to suppurative otitis media with offensive pus.
				In the tubercular miasm there may be eczematous eruptions and pustules about the ears, humid eruptions, incrustations and fissures (syphilo-tubercular).
3. Sensation	In psora there is constant itching, a sensation of crawling, dryness and pulsation in the ears.	Sycotic ears have stitching, pulsating, wandering pains.	Burning, bursting, and tearing ear pains are syphilitics.	The tubercular miasm has a sensation of flushing about the ears.
4. Modalities	The psoric patient cannot tolerate noise, due to over-sensitivity and many sounds cause pain in the ears.	Sycotic ear pains are aggravated during day and by changes in the weather.	Otitis media, with offensive discharge of pus is aggravated at night and from warmth.	Suppurative otitis media appearing in measles, chickenpox and scarlet fever when the fever is at its peak, indicates a good prognosis.
				Recurrent earache with swelling of the glands is aggravated at night and ameliorated during the daytime.

Key Word	Psoric Ear	Sycotic Ear	Syphilitic Ear	Tubercular Ear
5. Concomitant	Nervous restlessness and anxieties may accompany psoric ear symptoms.	In sycosis, pains in the ears make the patient physically restless.	Otitis media is a concomitant with the common cold, eruptions, measles, chicken pox etc. In syphilis, eczemas, which appear behind and about the ears, have thick, foetid pus and cracks.	There may be a peculiar carrion like odour from aural abscesses and any discharges are often cheesy or curdled. There may be eczematous eruptions around the ears, which are humid and pustular. Tonsillitis with earaches. Ears may look flushed and red. Even when there are foetid and copious discharges from the ears, the tubercular child feels alright and says that there is nothing the matter with him.
6. Hearing	The psoric patient has very sensitive hearing and is easily startled by noise.	Incoordination in the sense of hearing causes the patient to hear better in noisy places.	Impairment and total loss of hearing may occur in syphilis.	Loss of hearing with foetid, cheesy, curdled discharge from the ears.

MIASMATIC DIAGNOSIS:
<u>COMPARISON OF NASAL SYMPTOMS</u>

Key Word	Psoric Nose	Sycotic Nose	Syphilitic Nose	Tubercular Nose
1. Clinicals	Rhinitis.	Sinusitis.	Degenerative and ulcerative conditions of the nose.	Epistaxis.
		DNS (Deviated nasal septum).		Nasal polyps are tri-miasmatic.
		Swollen adenoids.		
2. Characteristics	In psora we find various olfactory disturbances of functional origin.	In sycosis, there are polyps, growths, moles, papilloma and veruccas in the nostrils. There may also be oedematous swelling of the nasal turbinate.	In syphilis, the nose may be flat or depressed from ulceration or destruction of the nasal septum and ulcers may occur inside the nostrils.	There is a tendency to the recurrent catching of colds in the tubercular miasm.
	Sensation of dryness in the nose.	Bland discharges with a fish-brine smell are characteristic of sycosis.	Clinkers (thick crusts which are dark green, black, or brown), can be offensive and often have to be removed. Manifest with offensive breath.	Epistaxis, which is bright red, may occur from any trivial cause such as over-heating or over-exercise or during fever. Relief comes by cold application but nose bleeds are difficult to stop and recur periodically.
	Psoric colds begin with sneezing, redness and heat. The nose becomes sensitive after it has been blown for some time.	Difficulty in breathing through the nose can be caused by various growths or oedema.		Flushing in the face, eyes and nose is tubercular.
	Discharges are thin and watery and can be acrid.	Moist snuffles with a purulent, scanty discharge with the odour of fish-brine and no formation of crust.		Snuffles are periodic and associated with haemorrhage.

Key Word	Psoric Nose	Sycotic Nose	Syphilitic Nose	Tubercular Nose
	Stoppage of one nostril causes mouth breathing.	Dr. Roberts suggests that sycotic nasal discharges are acrid and corrode the skin. However, acridity of discharges is generally syphilitic.		A thick yellowish discharge with an odour of old cheese or sulphur, ameliorated by cold application is constantly dropping down the throat (post nasal drip).
		There may be a mottled appearance of the mucus membrane.		Nasal polyps (which is tri-miasmatic) are termed as tubercular when characterised by profuse haemorrhage.
		Children born of sycotic parents complicated with gout, take cold easily at the slightest exposure and frequently suffer from acute, copious (+++) watery coryza, which is often excoriating.		Tubercular children haemorrhage from the nose from the least provocation. Blowing the nose, a slight knock, or even washing the face may initiate the nasal bleeding.
3. Modalities	Psoric nasal symptoms are aggravated in the morning, from cold and during sleep; and ameliorated from warmth and by natural discharges.	Sycotic nasal complaints are aggravated by damp and from changes in the weather. Amelioration is from abnormal discharges through various mucus membranes, such as coryza.	In syphilis, nasal symptoms are aggravated at night and from the warmth of the bed, and ameliorated by abnormal discharges.	In the tubercular miasm, nasal conditions are aggravated in a closed room and ameliorated in open air.
				Amelioration by epistaxis is also characteristic of the tubercular miasm.

Key Word	Psoric Nose	Sycotic Nose	Syphilitic Nose	Tubercular Nose
4. Smell	In psora we may find hypo-sensitivity to smell where the sense of smell is weak or lost, or an increased sense of smell due to hyper-susceptibility. Psoric patients often cannot tolerate any odours whether good or bad. At times they may become faint, and this hyper-sensitivity may even disturb their sleep; and can induce symptoms, such as nausea, vomiting and headaches.	Sycotic incoordination results in the sense of smell being increased profoundly or diminished.	The syphilitic sense of smell may be diminished, lost or perverted.	The tubercular sense of smell is characterised by changeableness and alternation. The patient will alternately smell through each nostril when the other is blocked.
5. Septum	Psora suffers from painful boils in the nose or pimples on the septum but there are no malignant manifestations. There is redness of the mucus membrane of the nasal orifice and a sooty, dirty appearance of the septum. In rhinitis, the septum is often dry, hot and burning.	In sycosis, burning of the nasal septum can lead to obstruction of the nose Thickening of the membranes or enlargement of the turbinate bones due to congestion may cause stoppages. Sycotic discharges are either yellow (also tubercular), greenish or greenish-yellow, except in fresh colds where there tends to be copious but thin mucus.	Recurrent boils in the nostrils may result in anosmia. Destruction of the septum is characteristic of the syphilitic miasm.	Tubercular nostrils are narrow and have small openings leading to nasal blockages and thereby mouth breathing.

Key Word	Psoric Nose	Sycotic Nose	Syphilitic Nose	Tubercular Nose
6. Hay Fever	Psoric hay fever is characterised by sneezing, redness and heat and by sensitiveness and a watery discharge.	In sycotic hay fever the discharge is scanty but the patient cannot breathe through the nose or blow any mucus from it. The slightest discharge however relieves the stopped up feeling.	Syphilitic discharges from hay fever are acrid, putrid and offensive.	Tubercular hay fever is periodic and recurrent with much sneezing and various allergic manifestations. The nose may feel clear one hour and be extremely stuffed-up the next. These cases are more difficult to cure and are often characterised by thick and occasionally blood-streaked discharges.

MIASMATIC DIAGNOSIS:
COMPARISON OF THE ORAL SYMPTOMS

Key Word	Psoric Mouth	Sycotic Mouth	Syphilitic Mouth	Tubercular Mouth
1. Clinicals	Stomatitis.	Salivary duct calculi.	Leucoplakia with fungal infection is syphilitic.	Haematemesis.
	Thrush.	Leucoplakia.		
2. Characteristics	Psora does not like to eat highly aromatic or strong smelling substances.	Tumours, warts and papillomas are characteristic of sycosis.	Syphilis is subject to various ulcers in the oral cavity.	In the tubercular miasm we may find various ulcers in the oral cavity, and bright red gums, which may bleed from the slightest touch.
	Ptyalism.		Oozing of blood from the gums, which often comes in the last stage of typhoid fever.	Salivation associated with recurrent hawking and clearing of the throat, due to a sensation of lodged mucus.
	Foetor oris.		Syphilitic saliva is ropy and can be drawn into long threads.	Foetor oris.
				Tonsillitis.
3. Taste (All of the miasms may experience either a partial or complete loss of taste.)	All food tastes 'as if burnt', is characteristic of psora. There may be various bad tastes in the mouth, either sourish, an intolerable sweet taste or a bitter taste which is often experienced in the open air.	Sycotic patients are subject to fishy, musty or putrid tastes.	In syphilis there is a metallic, especially coppery taste and the patient always has an unpleasant taste in the mouth.	In the tubercular miasm there is a taste of blood, frequently present in the morning, and of pus. There may also be an occasional bitter·where even water can taste unpleasant.

Key Word	Psoric Mouth	Sycotic Mouth	Syphilitic Mouth	Tubercular Mouth
	Perverseness of taste (psora-syphilitic) may occur in which for example, bread tastes bitter or water tastes unusual. Food may sometimes be rejected by the psoric patient who thinks that it tastes abnormal. Psoric eructations taste of recently eaten food or of fat.			Expectoration tastes sweetish, or salty or of rotten eggs, or may be devoid of taste altogether.
4. Tongue	In psora, there may be burning of the tongue and lips with swelling, or the tongue may be dry and coated or yellow with a bitter taste.	Warts and tumours may be visible on the tongue in sycosis.	In syphilis, imprints of the teeth are visible on the tongue. The tongue may be moist and emit a horribly offensive odour from mouth.	Glossitis is tubercular and there may be a whitish or yellowish coating to the tongue. Ulcers, which look like yoghurt or curd, may also be present.
5. Concomitants	Tartar and other improper substances lodge in the gums, tongue and root of the teeth.	Gum boils without pus formations are sycotic.	In syphilis, gumboils occur with the formation of pus, and there may be loose teeth with offensive saliva.	Tubercular oral symptoms may be associated with gum bleeding, tonsillitis and the recurrent catching of colds with coryza.
6. Teeth	Psoric teeth are painful and bleed easily. Pain from toothache may be intolerable.		Crowns of incisor teeth become crescent shaped. Syphilitic teeth are subject to pathological and structural changes in the dental arch. They are irregular in shape and in order of eruption.	Soft, spongy, receding gums are characteristic of the tubercular miasm. Teeth are irregular and bleed on slightest touch. They also decay as soon as they appear and may be deformed or asymmetrical.

Key Word	Psoric Mouth	Sycotic Mouth	Syphilitic Mouth	Tubercular Mouth
			Syphilitic children suffer every time a tooth comes through and diarrhoea, colds, tonsillitis etc, result.	Teething is painful and accompanied by diarrhoea (sycotic), spasms or convulsions (syphilo-tubercular) and digestive disturbances.
			Asymmetrical teeth, which are decayed and serrated; caries and dental fistulas are syphilitic.	The dental arch is imperfect or irregular.

MIASMATIC DIAGNOSIS:
COMPARISON OF THE FACIAL SYMPTOMS

Key Word	Psoric Face	Sycotic Face	Syphilitic Face	Tubercular Face
1. Characteristics	Usually the psoric face is devoid of perspiration, but conversely can show excessive perspiration.	Sycotic face is swollen and oedematous with reflections of the features of incoordination such as dermoid cysts, tumours and warts.	A greyish, greasy face is characteristic of this miasm and syphilitic children have ashy grey faces, the appearance of marasmus and the general look of a wrinkled, old man.	The tubercular face is characterised by sunken eyes and pallor although flushing of the cheeks appears during the evening. Rise of temperature with flushed face during attacks of cough and cold, during dentition or with wormy complaints.
2. General	Hot flushes to the face appear during the climacteric in the psoric miasm. There may be a hot feeling of the face, especially before periods and periodical hot flushes felt in the face, eyes and ears.	In sycosis, perspiration of the face has a fishy odour.	Syphilitic perspiration of the face and head is often seen as droplets. Syphilitic skin feels cool to touch.	In the tubercular miasm we find red spots on the cheeks with flushes of heat to the head and chest.
3. Appearance	The psoric face has dry, itching pimples and simple acne.	The sycotic face can be pale (psora-sycotic), bluish and dropsical.	In syphilis there is hard acne on the face.	Bloated (syco-tubercular) appearance of face, especially after sleep.

Key Word	Psoric Face	Sycotic Face	Syphilitic Face	Tubercular Face
	There may be a dry, rough, unwashed appearance.	In sycosis we also find a yellow, shallow, puffy, oedematous appearance.	The syphilitic appearance is of high check bones, thick lips and in some cases rough facial skin. The voice may be coarse and deep and is often hollow. The eyelids are red, inflamed and scaly with crusty, broken, stubby and irregularly curved lashes.	Paleness of the face is evident on rising in the morning or after sleep or eating. There may be a cyanotic, blue appearance and a look of anaemic especially as a result of prolonged or profuse haemorrhage.
	The shape of the psoric face is inverted.	Stubby, thick and broken hairs appear in the beard.	A flat, depressed nose is characteristic of syphilis.	Face and head is the shape of a pyramid with the apex at the chin.
	Pale and sallow, sometimes the eyes have a sunken appearance with blue rings (also tubercular).			The tubercular face can also be round, with fair, smooth, clear skin and a waxy complexion. The eyes are bright and sparkling and eyebrows and lashes are soft, glossy, long and silky. The nose is well shaped and the features sharp.
	The psoric patient may have a cyanotic, blue face and an anaemic appearance.			Recurrent, small, painful pimples and boils are characteristic of the tubercular miasm.
4. Lips	Psora has burning, itching lips, which may also be swollen.	In sycosis we find swollen lips with warts and veruccas.	In syphilis there is occasional redness of the lips (like tubercular).	Flushed, red lips, where the blood seems on the point of bursting.

Key Word	Psoric Face	Sycotic Face	Syphilitic Face	Tubercular Face
	Psoric lips are red or blue and congested in patients with poor circulation. Vesicles about the mouth are small, white and transparent, accompanied by much itching.		Deep fissures.	Deep fissures.
5. Facial Expression During Fever	Bright red and shining, and in cases of erysipelas, a sycotic element will also be present.	The sycotic face appears oedematous and heavy during fever.	During fever, syphilitic features are reflective of the dullness and morose feelings of the patient.	The tubercular face is usually pale with circumscribed red spots on the cheeks appearing in the afternoons or evenings in such conditions as dentition, worms, febrile states, colds etc.

MIASMATIC DIAGNOSIS:
<u>COMPARISON OF THE RESPIRATORY SYMPTOMS</u>

Key Word	Psoric Respiratory System	Sycotic Respiratory System	Syphilitic Respiratory System	Tubercular Respiratory System
1. Clinicals	Bronchitis (psora-tubercular).	Pneumonia with consolidation of the lungs.	Ulcerative sore throat.	Pleurisy.
	Pharyngitis.	Emphysema and fibrosis of the lungs.	Quinsy.	Pulmonary tuberculosis.
	Functional diseases of the respiratory system.	Vocal cord nodules.	Lung abscesses.	Tonsillitis, especially recurrent.
2. Structure	In psoric respiratory disorders, the natural curves of the chest remain unchanged.	In sycosis there is an oedematous appearance of the nose, uvula and tonsils with hypertrophy of the nasal turbinate.	In syphilis, there may be a flat, depressed appearance of the nose and irregular depressions in the chest cavity related to collapse of the lungs.	The tubercular chest is often narrow and lacking in width laterally, and in depth antero-posteriorly. The sub-clavicular spaces are hollow.
			Ulcers may be present in the respiratory passage, nose, tonsils and trachea.	The sternum is thin, and flat on the top but protrudes at the lower end and the xiphoid process giving it a barrel shaped appearance — pigeon chest.
			Ulceration, cavities and abscesses may be found especially in advanced lung conditions.	Tubercular shoulders are often rounded and incline forwards infringing on the chest area.
				One lung is larger and better developed than the other, resulting in hyper-functioning of that lung.

Key Word	Psoric Respiratory System	Sycotic Respiratory System	Syphilitic Respiratory System	Tubercular Respiratory System
				Curves and lines in the chest wall are imperfect and certain areas may be sunken and depressed.
3. Sensation	The psoric patient experiences burning pains in the chest and the sensation of a band around the chest.	In sycosis there is a feeling of stitching pains in chest with different types of aching ameliorated by pressure.	Syphilis experiences rawness and soreness in the throat and tonsils.	In the tubercular miasm there is a sensation of mucus constantly stuck in the throat, accompanied by tickling.
4. Location	Psoric respiratory infections generally occur in the upper respiratory tract. There is recurrent catching of colds, and the nose and throat are sensitive.	Sycotic features of incoordination include dilatation of the bronchi and bronchioles as well as the lungs.	Syphilitic respiratory symptoms can manifest anywhere in the respiratory passage, from the nose down to the lung alveoli with features of ulceration, destruction, cavity formation and pyogenic inflammation.	The tubercular patient catches cold easily and therefore always covers up their throat and chest warmly.
5. Modality	All psoric respiratory complaints are aggravated during the winter and from cold, and are ameliorated by warmth in general and the appearance of natural discharges.	Sycotic asthma, pneumonia, bronchitis and coughs and colds are all aggravated in humid moist atmospheres, from changes in the season and during rainy spells.	The syphilitic patient feels worse at night and during the morning.	Aggravation of tubercular respiratory complaints comes from cold air and from milk (which builds up lots of catarrh). Symptoms are also worse at night.
		Asthma with profuse expectoration, which is aggravated in the early morning, is characterised by the patient's compulsion to move about. Amelioration comes from lying on the abdomen.		Amelioration is from open air and epistaxis.

Key Word	Psoric Respiratory System	Sycotic Respiratory System	Syphilitic Respiratory System	Tubercular Respiratory System
		Asthma (bronchospasm) is ameliorated by passing stool.		
6. Concomitants	Anxiety and apprehension of incurable diseases, even when the patient is suffering from trivial ailments, is a characteristic of psora.	Restlessness accompanies sycosis — the patient likes to be constantly on the move.	Dysphagia and dyspnoea are syphilitic manifestations but can also be mixed miasmatic. A pus-like putrid expectoration may accompany a syphilitic cough.	Along with tubercular coughs and colds, there is always swelling of the tonsils and of the glands around the neck (cervical lymphadenopathy).
				There is a great sense of exhaustion and the patient tires easily even after sleep. They feel better and regain their strength as the day advances or the sun ascends but weaken again as the sun goes down.
7. Voice	In psora there is huskiness of the voice with dryness of the throat.		Hoarseness occurs in syphilis especially before menstruation.	Voice is coarse and deep with base-like chest tones. There may also be a 'croak' in the voice.
8. Cough	The psoric patient suffers from a dry spasmodic cough resulting from suppression of measles, skin disease etc. which causes the lungs to be affected.	The coughs of sycotics are usually bronchial.	In syphilis we find a short, barking cough. There may be just one or two distinct barks like that of a dog.	The cough of the tubercular patient is deep and prolonged, giving us the lower chest tones. It is worse in the morning and when the patient first lies down in the evening.
	In psora, the cough is dry, teasing and spasmodic in type.	Hard, racking coughs often in early winter also affect the sycotic patient.	The syphilitic cough may also be paroxysmal.	Teasing cough (which indicates the weakness of the lungs).

Key Word	Psoric Respiratory System	Sycotic Respiratory System	Syphilitic Respiratory System	Tubercular Respiratory System
		A great deal of coughing is required to raise even a tiny amount of mucus; hence the cough is prolonged and teasing.		Quite often the cough of the tubercular patient is deep, ringing and hollow with no expectoration. Tubercular coughs are often so dry and tight that they induce headache or the whole body is shaken by their explosive paroxysms.
9. Expectoration	In psora we find haemoptysis, as a result of functional disturbances of the lungs. However, prolonged and persistent haemoptysis can only be possible if the tubercular miasm is present.	The coughs of sycosis have very little expectoration, although there is a large accumulation of mucus in the lungs (this is a feature of incoordination, i.e. large accumulation but little expectoration).	The syphilitic paroxysmal cough is accompanied by a tasteless yellowish/greenish or clear, sticky thread-like discharge.	Mucus, which is viscid, pus-like, sticky, musty or offensive and tastes sweetish or salty, and may sometimes be mixed with blood, is a characteristic indication of the tubercular miasm.
	There is frequent congestion of the throat with the accumulation of much phlegm.	The mucus is usually yellowish or clear (when clear white mucus is expectorated, then the psoric component is also present).		Tubercular expectoration always sinks down and cannot float. It is purulent, greenish-yellow and very often offensive.
	The psoric patient usually expectorates mucus, which is scanty and tasteless.			The tubercular miasms shows a constant desire to hawk or clear the throat from a viscid, scanty mucus.

Key Word	Psoric Respiratory System	Sycotic Respiratory System	Syphilitic Respiratory System	Tubercular Respiratory System
10. Respiration	Psoric respiration is slow and sallow.	In sycosis we find tachypnoea, i.e. accelerated/rapid respiration.	Dyspnoea before going to bed, or while lying down is indicative of the syphilitic miasm.	In the tubercular miasm, dyspnoea is apparent on ascending stairs. There is weakness and debility, and the breathlessness is often painful.
	As psoric symptoms are characterised by 'hypo' or less, scanty and absence, so the features of hypoxia, anoxia and anoxaemia are classified as psoric manifestations.			Tubercular patients are poor breathers, which results in laboured respiration. They have no desire to take a full breath even though there may be no obstructions in the air passages. As a consequence, the alveoli of the lungs are never fully expanded and do not receive adequate oxygen causing atrophies and the walls to glue together. This can be linked to a dislike of taking in cold air, for fear of being chilled or catching cold.
	Babies which are born pale and cyanosed and in need of resuscitation, due to defective oxygenation and hypoxia caused by the umbilical cord being around the neck during intra-uterine life, can be rescued by treatment from anti-psoric medicines.			The tubercular patient is unable to expand the chest fully as the expansive power of the lungs is greatly limited.

Key Word	Psoric Respiratory System	Sycotic Respiratory System	Syphilitic Respiratory System	Tubercular Respiratory System
11. **Associated Symptoms**	In psora there may be frequent stitches in the chest with or without cough.	Sycosis has nasal blockages; and the patient is generally unable to breathe through the nose.	In syphilis, there are destructive changes in the lung parenchyma, lung abscesses, and collapse of the lungs. Advanced pathological changes in the lungs may also occur.	Even with advanced lung conditions, tubercular patients are full of hopes and will never concede that the disease is incurable. They are also likely to say that there is nothing the matter with them. Headache alternates with chest complaints. Cough can induce headache. Glandular swelling and changes in the cervical region may precede lung changes.

MIASMATIC DIAGNOSIS:
COMPARISON OF THE CARDIAC SYMPTOMS

Key Word	Psoric Heart	Sycotic Heart	Syphilitic Heart	Tubercular Heart
1. Clinicals	In psora, cardiac and emotional symptoms alternate (for alternation of symptoms in a recurrent way the tubercular miasm has to be present).	In sycosis, the heart is affected as a result of suppression of rheumatic complaints.	· The syphilitic patient is liable to suffer from ulcerative bacterial endocarditis, and heart affections with valvular degeneration.	Palpitations, and a rush of blood to the head and chest with redness of the face and flushed cheeks is characteristic of the tubercular miasm.
	Heart affections may occur from fear, disappointment, loss of friends and over-excitement.	Sycosis has incoordination (such as mitral or aortic regurgitation), dilatation and abnormality of the cardiac valves. RHD (rheumatic heart diseases). Hypertrophy of the heart, and left or right ventricular hypertrophy of the heart.	Syphilis is also subject to congenital abnormalities such as Fallot's tetralogy and PDA (Patent Ductus Arteriosus), which are the cause of structural and/or developmental anomalies.	
	Psoric cardiac symptoms are mostly of a functional nature and accompanied by great anxiety and fear of incurable disease or death.	Sycotic patients are generally fleshy and puffy and their dyspnoea is caused by obesity.		
	Anxiety about the heart with constant worry typifies psora.	A combination of sycosis and psora creates the right soil for valvular and cardiac disturbances.		

Key Word	Psoric Heart	Sycotic Heart	Syphilitic Heart	Tubercular Heart
2. Sensation	In psora, there is a feeling of increased circulatory function, congestion and plethora. The precordium may either feel empty or heavy.	In sycosis pain radiates from the precordium to the shoulder or scapular region or vice versa.	In syphilis there is a sensation of heaviness in the precordium with a lack of expression.	Violent palpitations with beating and shaking (for shaking of the frame the sycotic miasm may be present) of the whole body is representative of the tubercular miasm.
	There may be a hammering sensation in the region of the heart, and many other uncomfortable sensations.	Sycotic cardiac pains are like an electric shock, which comes and goes suddenly.		
	The psoric patient may experience a violent rush of blood (in which case the tubercular miasm is likely to be present) to the chest, and a sensation of weakness, goneness, soreness or fullness around the heart.	Soreness or tenderness around the precordium is made worse by the motion of the arms.		
	Sharp, cutting, piercing neuralgic pains about the heart, pulsations of the heart which shake the whole body, and a sensation as if there were a band around the heart are also typical of the psoric miasm.	Sycosis suffers from fluttering, throbbing with oppression and difficulty in breathing at intervals.		

Key Word	Psoric Heart	Sycotic Heart	Syphilitic Heart	Tubercular Heart
3. Modalities	In psora, all heart complaints including cardiac pains and angina are aggravated in the evening, from movement, from coughing, laughing, and after eating. The stitching pains (with which there is generally a sycotic component) of angina almost kill the patient when they make any attempt at movement.	Heat and changes in the weather aggravate sycotic heart conditions.	Syphilitic cardiac problems are aggravated at night, from sunset, perspiration, and extremes of temperature, movement and from the warmth of the bed.	The tubercular patient suffering from a heart condition wants to keep still. They are aggravated by higher altitudes and cannot climb stairs or ascend hills. Breathing on ascending is difficult and sitting up causes the patient to feel dizzy and faint. Aggravation also comes from pressure on the chest and at night.
	Oppression and feelings of anxiety are worse in the morning.	Amelioration is from gentle exercise such as slow walking or riding, except in conditions of rheumatic origin where motion aggravates.	Amelioration occurs during the day (from sunrise to sunset), from changes of position and from cold in general.	Tubercular conditions are ameliorated by lying down and in open air.
	Psoric cardiac symptoms are ameliorated by eructation, and from rest and lying down.	All sorts of abnormal discharges ameliorate and are of good prognostic value in sycosis.		
4. Concomitants	The psoric patient always thinks the heart's action is about to stop and that he will die soon. He keeps his mind on his heart, and is constantly taking his own pulse.	Dyspnoea with pain about the heart; gout and rheumatism of the heart are sycotic manifestations.	Palpitations, which are tuberculo-syphilitic, occur.	Tubercular heart troubles are accompanied by fainting, temporary loss of vision, ringing in the ears, pallor and great weakness.
	In psora, heart problems are accompanied by much anxiety, mental distress, depression and sadness.	Marked anasarca and dropsical manifestations such as cardiac dropsy occur. (Some authors suggest this to be syco-psoric). Gout and rheumatism of the heart are sycotic manifestations.		There is a constant but gradual 'falling away of the chest' and a rush of blood to the chest and face in tubercular conditions.

Key Word	Psoric Heart	Sycotic Heart	Syphilitic Heart	Tubercular Heart
5. Pulse	Bradycardia is psoric.	Tachycardia is sycotic.	Irregularity in the pulse is syphilitic. This irregularity can be in rate or rhythm.	The tubercular pulse is feeble but rapid.
	The psoric pulse is full and bounding.	The sycotic pulse is slow and feeble, soft (for soft pulse a psoric component is also present) and easily compressible. The pulse lacks tension.		A small, thread-like but quick pulse is typical of the tubercular miasm.
6. Manifestations	Psoric dyspnoea is painful with features of cyanosis.	Thrombosis (where sycosis is mainly, but not always responsible), embolism (a feature of incoordination) and myocardial infarctions are sycotic. In a cardiac attack, there is imbalance and incoordination in the circulation associated with the formation of embolus or thrombus and sycosis is mainly responsible.	Syphilitics may have had heart troubles for years with occasional dyspnoea and pains, which they usually deny. They can drop dead suddenly however from massive cardiac failure (generally sycosis plays a role here too).	Tubercular dyspnoea is often painful.
		In sycosis there may be dropsical swelling and flabbiness after prolonged suffering from cardiac or respiratory complications.	Due to lack of expression and realisation, syphilitics do not convey their troubles to their friends, family or doctor.	
		There is seldom much pain or suffering in sycotic manifestations unless they are combined with rheumatic difficulties.		Persistent emaciation occurs in tubercular cardiac patients.

MIASMATIC DIAGNOSIS:
COMPARISON OF THE STOMACH SYMPTOMS

Key Word	Psoric Stomach	Sycotic Stomach	Syphilitic Stomach	Tubercular Stomach
1. Clinicals	Gastritis, oesophagitis with burning, and other functional disorders of the gastro-intestinal tract are psoric.	Meat arouses the latent sycosis and stimulates the formation of uric acid. It is therefore better for the sycotic patient to take meat sparingly and consume more nuts, beans or cheeses as a source of protein.	Ulcers and degenerative types of cancer result from the syphilitic miasm.	Gastro-intestinal disturbances such as haematemesis and melaena where bleeding predominates typify the tubercular miasm.
	Psora also has acidity, sour eructation, heartburn and nausea with a feeling of faintness.	In sycosis there are benign and encapsulated tumours, papilloma and polyps of the gastro-intestinal tract.		Milk allergies and allergies to different types of food are tubercular.
2. Sensations & Hunger	Empty, all-gone sensation, especially in the morning, as the patient is unable to assimilate any nutritious substances from the food they eat.	Crampy, colicky pains are sycotic. Children born of sycotic parents often suffer from colic from the moment of birth or colic may be initiated after vaccination.	In syphilis there are burning, bursting, tearing and ulcerative pains in the gastro-intestinal tract.	The tubercular patient feels like fainting if hunger is not quickly satisfied. Extreme hunger is associated with an all-gone, weak, empty feelings in the stomach (this from the psoric component of the miasm).
	The psoric patient may have an excessive hunger for unnatural substances like chalk, clay and other indigestible things especially during fever or pregnancy.	Three month colic in children who become restless, writhe, twist and squirm with pain and draw up the limbs.		In the tubercular miasm, patients are constantly hungry and eat beyond their capacity (this is from the sycotic component of the miasm) to digest, or they may have no appetite in morning but feel hungry for other meals.

Morbid and unnatural hunger (syphilitic component may be present) even after a full meal and at night while sleeping, as if the patient cannot be satiated. Cannot wait for a meal. Hungry especially between 10 a.m. and 11 a.m. The patient has to eat at once or else they become faint.

Psoric patients mostly eat beyond their capacity of digestion, which causes various types of diarrhoea, or the patient may be hungry but a few mouthfuls fill them up to the throat.

The psoric patient suffers from feelings of distension due to an accumulation of gas, with flatulence, rumbling and gurgling; and sour and bitter eructations which taste of the food just eaten. There is a sensation of fullness, weight and heaviness as if there is a stone or lump in the stomach.

All symptoms of acidity and dyspepsia, nausea and vomiting, and pains in the liver and stomach are psoric.

Key Word	Psoric Stomach	Sycotic Stomach	Syphilitic Stomach	Tubercular Stomach
	There may be a constant gnawing at the pit of the stomach with a cold or hot sensation. Beating, throbbing, constriction and oppression occur especially after eating.			
3. Modalities	In psora, aggravation occurs a few hours after eating. There is aggravation from protein and from being touched, and even the slightest pressure cannot be endured.	Sycotic patients are likely to suffer some discomfort after eating.	Syphilitics are aggravated at night, from extremes of temperature, warmth, and starch.	Tubercular patients suffer aggravation from milk, greasy and oily foods, at night, from any pressure on chest or stomach, and in closed rooms.
	Bilious nausea and vomiting which comes on at regular intervals is ameliorated by rest, quiet and sleep.	Aggravation comes from consuming meat and fat, and it is therefore better to restrict the consumption of meat in rheumatic patients.		Amelioration comes in the open air and in dry weather.
	Temporarily better after eating, but after some time the psoric patient will feel the distension, heaviness and other symptoms return and become aggravated.	In sycosis, amelioration is from lying on the stomach, violent motion, rocking (in case of children), walking, and hot food and drinks.		
	Psoric stomach complaints are generally ameliorated by hot food and drinks, belching and gentle motion.			
4. Concomitants	Shortness of breath, vertigo, giddiness, sweat and anxiety are associated with most psoric gastric symptoms.	Sycosis has loud eructation especially with colicky symptoms.	In syphilis, dullness and depression are associated with gastric manifestations.	In the tubercular miasm, a red face and flushed chin accompany gastric complaints.

Key Word	Psoric Stomach	Sycotic Stomach	Syphilitic Stomach	Tubercular Stomach
	In psora, headaches, weariness and sleepiness come on after eating.			Swelling of the intestinal and mesenteric glands may also occur.
5. Cravings	In psora we find craving for certain items or foods, which are refused when, offered, especially in children.	Sycotics (like syphilitics) crave alcohol and tend to abuse it. Beer is preferred as it causes less aggravation than wine.	Syphilitic patients have a perverted craving for alcohol.	Tubercular patients are characterised by a craving for peculiar foods and foods which make them sick.
	Craving for sweet things is followed by vomiting of bile.	There is a craving for rich gravies, table salt, pungent and salty foods, and cold or hot foods.	There may be a craving for cold food.	Meat, potatoes and salt are also craved and salt may be eaten straight from the saucer.
	During fever the psoric patient may have an aversion to sweets and crave acids instead. They may also crave greasy and highly seasoned foods and meat but these do not suit them.			Tubercular patients are extremists and like foods to be either really hot or really cold.
	There is a craving for stimulants such as tea, coffee and tobacco to supply the nerve force.			
	A craving for unusual things during pregnancy but which goes off after the birth, may sometimes be passed onto the child.			

Key Word	Psoric Stomach	Sycotic Stomach	Syphilitic Stomach	Tubercular Stomach
6. Desires	In psora there is a desire for sweets, acids, pickles, sour and indigestible things, meat, ghee (butter oil), hot, spicy and oily foods.	Sycotics desire warm food, coconut and betelnut etc.	As the syphilitic miasm vitiates the mind leading to a lack of expression and realisation; any striking desires and aversions cannot be properly ascertained.	Tubercular patients desire foods, which aggravates their condition. They have an inability to assimilate much starch.
	Psoric patients want everything fried if possible and have a strong repugnance to boiled foods.	Sycotic patients like fat meat well seasoned with salt and pepper and served with rich gravies.	The syphilitic tendency for destruction leads to a desire for stimulants such as tea, coffee, tobacco and wine. There may be a hereditary tendency to alcoholism. Syphilitic patients suffer from nervous weakness and generally feel better for stimulants.	A desire for too warm or too cold food is tubercular and patients thrive better on fat and fat foods. They require plenty of salt and do not easily digest starches.
	A desire for fats, greasy foods, rich pastries and sweet-meats, when satisfied can induce bilious attacks.	A desire for beer is sycotic.	There are desires for very spicy meat (dislikes less spicy preparations), for cold food and drinks, lime and sweet and sour foods. The syphilitic patient also desires milk, which they are unable to assimilate, and indigestible things like chalk, slate, pencil and wine.	There is a longing for stimulants such as beer and wine, and for hot, aromatic foods.

Key Word	Psoric Stomach	Sycotic Stomach	Syphilitic Stomach	Tubercular Stomach
7. Aversions	Psoric patients have both an aversion to and an intolerance of milk. They are also averse to boiled and cold foods.	In sycosis we find an intolerance of spices and aversions to milk and meat. (With regards to meat, there are two different opinions — some authors believe that sycotic patients like fatty meats, and my own belief is that they like meat but that it does not like them). Aversion and/or aggravation from green leafy vegetables; spinach, onion, juicy fruits etc. Any fruit or vegetable, which has a high water content, aggravates the hydrogenoid, sycotic constitution.	The syphilitic patient has a complete aversion to meat and to animal foods.	Milk allergies are present in the tubercular miasm and patients cannot tolerate milk in any form. As the tubercular miasm is changeable, there is a possibility of a strong desire or aversion to rich gravies. Cravings are for potatoes and meat.

MIASMATIC DIAGNOSIS:
COMPARISON OF THE ABDOMINAL SYMPTOMS

Key Word	Psoric Abdomen	Sycotic Abdomen	Syphilitic Abdomen	Tubercular Abdomen
1. Clinicals	Duodenitis, cholecystitis, non-functioning of the gall bladder, colitis and other inflammations of the abdomen, mainly of functional origin and including gastric refluxes are of psoric origin. Ascitis is syco-psoric.	Tumours, papillomas and encapsulated malignant growths in the abdomen and cholelithiasis (gallstones) are sycotic.	Degeneration of the liver cells, including fatty degeneration is of syphilitic origin.	In the tubercular miasm we find swelling of the intestinal and mesenteric glands.
	Constipation is primarily psoric.	Diarrhoea is sycotic (characterised by exaggerated peristalsis).	Dysentery is syphilitic (characterised by irregular peristalsis).	Breakfast diarrhoea or diarrhoea after eating and stool with blood (melaena) is tubercular.
	Dyspeptic symptoms are also psoric in origin.	Appendicitis and appendicular colic are always sycotic.	Cirrhosis of the liver is syphilo-sycotic, as there is incoordination as well as degeneration of the liver cells.	Hernia has a strong psoric element as laxation of the muscles is due to psora but recurrence or persistence is due to the tubercular miasm.
		In children, swelling and protrusion of the umbilicus with a thin, yellowish-green discharge and the odour of fish-brine is characteristic of sycosis.		In tubercular children we find recurrent ulceration of the umbilicus with a yellow discharge.
		Hepato or hepato-splenomegaly (either liver enlargement or liver and spleen enlargement).		Lymphatic involvement of the abdomen is tubercular.

Key Word	Psoric Abdomen	Sycotic Abdomen	Syphilitic Abdomen	Tubercular Abdomen
2. Sensation	Sore, bruised, pressive pains in the abdomen are psoric. In psora there are sensations of heaviness, fullness with distension of the abdomen; heartburn and waterbrash. There may also be a bearing down sensation. An empty, all-gone feeling is characteristic of psora. There may be a stuffed up feeling, which prevents eating, or the psoric patient may experience a sensation of constriction in the abdomen. Rumbling and gurgling occurs in the abdomen as soon as the psoric patient eats or drinks.	Stitching, pulsating and wandering pains in the abdomen are sycotic.	The syphilitic patient is subject to burning, bursting and tearing sensations in the abdomen. The stool may contain scrapings of intestine or jelly-like lumps of mucus.	Tubercular patients can feel the beating of the abdominal aorta through the abdominal walls. The tubercular abdomen is saucer shaped or may resemble a large plate turned bottom side up.
3. Characteristics	Slow peristalsis is psoric. Stitches on stooping or bending the body.	Accelerated and exaggerated intestinal peristalsis is sycotic. In sycosis, colic is produced by the simplest of foods.	Dysenteric spasm, especially at night, drives the patient out of bed and may be associated with profuse debilitating perspiration. Perverted intestinal peristalsis resulting dysentery is syphilitic.	In the tubercular miasm we find colic of the lower abdomen, rumbling and gurgling, and flatulence, which causes lower abdominal pain.

Key Word	Psoric Abdomen	Sycotic Abdomen	Syphilitic Abdomen	Tubercular Abdomen
		Children born of sycotic parents often suffer from colic almost from the moment of birth.		
4. Modalities	All psoric complaints but especially those of the abdomen are aggravated after eating which causes bloating. The patient cannot bear anything to touch the abdomen.	In sycosis, abdominal pains compel the patient to bend forward.	Syphilitics are aggravated at night and from warmth.	Tubercular patients experience aggravation from milk and fruits, and from greasy and oily foods.
	Cramps in abdomen from potatoes and beans.	Crampy colicky, spasmodic pains, which come on in paroxysms, are ameliorated by hard pressure.	Amelioration for syphilitic abdominal pains is from cold.	Aggravation may also occur when pressure is applied to the abdomen.
	Psoric pains in the abdomen are ameliorated by heat and by gentle pressure, in which case the sycotic miasm must also be present.			Amelioration is from the open air.

64

MIASMATIC DIAGNOSIS:
<u>COMPARISON OF THE RECTAL SYMPTOMS</u>

Key Word	Psoric Rectum	Sycotic Rectum	Syphilitic Rectum	Tubercular Rectum
1. Clinicals	Constipation.	Prolapse of the rectum.	Perineal pyogenic inflammations (perineal abscess).	Rectal haemorrhage.
	Morning diarrhoeas.	Diarrhoeas and any stool where colic predominates.	Dysentery with blood and pus.	Bloody stool and early morning diarrhoeas.
			IBS (irritable bowel syndrome) where pus and mucus in the stool predominate.	IBS (irritable bowel syndrome) where blood predominates.
		Blind and non-bleeding haemorrhoids and polyps.		Bleeding haemorrhoids and polyps.
			Fistulas and abscesses.	Recurrent rectal fistulas and abscesses.
				Worms of various types.
2. Characteristics	Constipation is primarily psoric but in psora we may also find morning diarrhoeas.	Diarrhoea is sycotic.	All types of pyogenic inflammations of the rectum are syphilitic.	Bleeding from rectum is characteristic of the tubercular miasm.
		The sycotic stool is sour, grass green in colour and may be accompanied by constant, gripping colic.	In syphilis, the stool may contain scrapings of intestine or jelly-like lumps of mucus.	Alternation of rectal diseases with heart, chest or lung troubles, especially asthma or respiratory difficulties. Sometimes tubercular manifestations of the brain alternate with bowel difficulties.

Key Word	Psoric Rectum	Sycotic Rectum	Syphilitic Rectum	Tubercular Rectum
		Colic accompanies diarrhoea. The greater the colic, the greater the sycosis.		
		Prolapse of the rectum is an incoordination and laxation of the muscles and is therefore syco-psoric (sycosis affords the incoordination and psora is responsible for ataxia or laxity of the muscles).		
3. Sensation	Soreness in the rectum and sore, bruised, pressive pains are characteristic of psora.	In sycosis we find stitching pains with pulsating sensations in the rectum.	Syphilis has burning and bursting sensations in the rectum.	In the tubercular miasm there is a sensation of portal congestion with heat and flushing in and around the rectum.
4. Modalities	Psoric diarrhoea can occur from fright, bad news or from preparation for an unusual ordeal, and is aggravated in the morning.	Sycotic diarrhoea is aggravated by changes in the weather, by cold and from getting wet. It is also worse from eating fruits.	Syphilitics are aggravated at night from warmth and ameliorated by cold.	Tubercular diarrhoeas are aggravated at night, or in the early morning, driving the patient out of bed. Cold, milk, meat, potatoes, fruits, greasy and oily foods also aggravate.
	Stool is worse from cold, slightest exposure, motion, and eating, especially over-eating, and drinking, particularly cold things.	In young children where diarrhoea is accompanied by colic, the child will want to be rocked or carried constantly.		The least exposure to cold brings on diarrhoea in tubercular children. Diarrhoea may also be aggravated or precipitated from teething.

Key Word	Psoric Rectum	Sycotic Rectum	Syphilitic Rectum	Tubercular Rectum
	Psoric rectal symptoms are ameliorated by pressure and warmth. They are better for warm drinks and hot food, and from warm applications to the abdomen.	Amelioration comes from lying on the abdomen or by pressing the lower abdomen.		
5. Concomitants	In psora, throbbing in the abdomen accompanies rectal pain.	Intestinal colic makes the sycotic patient restless and irritable.	Syphilitic rectal symptoms are associated with depression and melancholia.	In the tubercular miasm we find diarrhoea with profuse warm or cold debilitating perspiration.
	Constipation with pain in remote regions, such as the liver or head and associated with drowsiness, sleepiness and heaviness with no desire to work. Can also be associated with foul breath, coated tongue, nausea and loss of appetite.		Prolonged constipation may be associated with headache.	Tubercular children suffering from such diarrhoeas, may develop sudden brain stasis.
	Great weakness after diarrhoeiac stool.			Vomiting and retching may occur before stool.
6. Stool	Diarrhoea from gluttony (syco-psoric).	Sycotic diarrhoea can be corrosive and grassy-green. It may be accompanied by great pruritus and there is often a fish-brine smell.	Lienteria (diarrhoea in which the stool contains undigested food particles), diarrhoea and dysentery occur as syphilis perverts proper functioning of the digestive system and powers.	Tubercular children often cannot digest cow's milk in any form which results in undigested, curdled particles in the diarrhoeiac stool.

Key Word	Psoric Rectum	Sycotic Rectum	Syphilitic Rectum	Tubercular Rectum
	Painless diarrhoea due to fright.	With sycotic diarrhoea, the stool gushes and ejaculates forcefully. There is a jet-like expulsion of the faeces, with crampy pain. Colic may also be present.	Diarrhoea, which occurs at the seaside, is syphilitic.	Diarrhoea throughout dentition.
	Painless, offensive morning diarrhoea accompanied by rumbling and gurgling in the abdomen, may occur after taking cold things.	Pain in the rectum with diarrhoea, which may lead to the crying out of the patient. They may rush to the toilet due to a sense of insecurity.	Recurrent problems during the period of dentition lead to coughs and colds followed by diarrhoea and dysentery. There is then a further stage of scrofulous swelling of the glands leading to weakness and debility followed by watery diarrhoea, which mimics cholera.	Blood in the stool is a characteristic of the tubercular miasm.
	Obstipation (obstinate constipation), hard stool with no desire for defecation for a couple of days, or an ineffectual urge for defecation can be present.	Tenesmus in rectum with slimy, mucussy stool. Stool can also be sticky.	In syphilis we find extreme weakness from loose motion, and cholera infantum, which almost completely drains the system.	Many of the obstinate constipations come under the heading of this miasm.
	The psoric stool may be of any colour, and is generally watery and offensive. When passed, it may contain undigested food particles and is unlikely to be painful.	The sycotic stool is polychromatic, changeable (when characterised by incoordination), usually greenish-yellow and can be watery and sour smelling. Acidic stool, which corrodes the rectum (here acidity is the syphilitic component).	The syphilitic stool is black and extremely offensive. It may contain scrapings of intestine and shreds of mucus.	Greenish, bloody stool which may be copious and painless. Can be yellowish in colour (although generally yellow is the colour of sycosis, so this may denote mixed miasmatic tendencies), ashy or grey showing a lack of bile.

Key Word	Psoric Rectum	Sycotic Rectum	Syphilitic Rectum	Tubercular Rectum
				The tubercular stool is offensive, slimy, and bloody and may have a musty or mouldy smell. or an odour reminiscent of rotten eggs.
7. Worms	Worm symptoms are generally tuberculo-psoric, but when associated with irritation, grinding of the teeth, crawling, creeping and itching of the nose and rectum, then the manifestation is purely psoric. Thread worms.	Wormy symptoms with severe abdominal colic; hyperactive restlessness; excessive dribbling of saliva, and twitching of the muscles are indicative of incoordinations and are syco-psoric in origin.	Convulsions from worms are a syphilitic manifestation.	All varieties of wormy manifestations are generally recurrent which is characteristic of the tubercular miasm. They may also be associated with allergic manifestations, even allergic dermatitis. Pinworms and many other varieties of intestinal worms are tubercular.
8. Haemorrhoids	Haemorrhoids are generally syco-psoric and are classed under the psoric miasm when they are associated with discomfort and itching.	Rectal haemorrhoids with extreme sensitiveness and pain are sycotic.	Rectal fissures and haemorrhoids with putrid and foetid discharges are syphilitic. They may also ooze pus and sanious fluids.	Strictures, haemorrhoids, sinuses, fistulas and pockets in the rectum are all of tubercular origin and are much aggravated when combined with sycosis and syphilis. Cancerous rectal symptoms are a combinations of the tubercular and sycotic miasms. Bleeding haemorrhoids are tubercular. In this miasm, haemorrhoids, which are suppressed or operated on, may result in asthma-like lung difficulties or heart troubles.

Key Word	Psoric Urinary Symptoms	Sycotic Urinary Symptoms	Syphilitic Urinary Symptoms	Tubercular Urinary Symptoms
1. Clinical	Enuresis of functional origin is psoric.	Nephroblastoma, tumours of the kidneys, papillomas of the bladder and nephrotic syndrome where oedema predominates are sycotic.	Destructive and degenerative types of malignant tumours in the kidneys or bladder are syphilitic.	Enuresis, diabetes mellitus (generally tri-miasmatic) and diabetes insipidus (syco-tubercular).
	Nephritis, pyelitis, cystitis and urethritis are psoric in origin because of their infective nature (as all inflammation begins with psora) but strongly sycotic in their manifestations.	Sycosis also has renal dropsy, renal calculi and calculous deposits in other parts of the genito-urinary tract.	Pyaemia with oozing of pus.	Polyps and papillomas of the bladder with haemorrhage are tubercular.
		Hypertrophy of the prostate, and prostatitis from sexual over-indulgence.	Stricture of the urethra.	Haematuria.
2. Characteristics	Phosphaturia after febrile complications occurs in the psoric miasm.	Calculi, complications of the genito-urinary tract and various pains of the urinary tract are generally sycotic in manifestation.	All advanced conditions of the kidneys and genito-urinary tract, with pyogenic inflammations can be associated with structural and pathological changes, and are therefore syphilitic in origin.	The tubercular miasm is responsible for the production of haematuria resulting from different types of pathological manifestations of KUB (kidney, ureter and bladder):
	After fevers and acute diseases, the deposit in the urine is white or yellowish white.			Diabetes mellitus and enuresis are secondary symptoms of the tuberculo-psoric diathesis.

Key Word	Psoric Urinary Symptoms	Sycotic Urinary Symptoms	Syphilitic Urinary Symptoms	Tubercular Urinary Symptoms
	Anuria, oliguria, and stoppage or scanty urine from fright, tension or becoming chilled are psoric manifestations.			
3. Sensation	Psoric patients, especially those advancing in age, experience a sensation of fullness in the bladder. There may also be a feeling of constriction. Smarting and burning in the urinary meatus or in the lumbar area unrelated to any pathological causes might be present.	Stitching and pulsating sensations with wandering pains are sycotic.	Burning and bursting sensations in the bladder or loin area are syphilitic.	A tickling sensation in the urethra is characteristic of the tubercular miasm.
4. Modalities	Psora experiences aggravation from cold. Amelioration of psoric urinary symptoms comes from natural discharges such as urination.	Sycotic urinary symptoms are aggravated in damp, rainy weather and from the changes of the season.	All symptoms of syphilis are aggravated at night, in summer, and from warmth.	Tubercular urinary manifestations are aggravated at night. Amelioration is from the open air.
5. Concomitants	Psoric urinary problems may be associated with anxiety, apprehension and fear of incurable diseases.	Diabetes and albuminuria are tubercular, yet if the conditions are extremely severe, sycosis may also be present, and they can become tri-miasmatic.	In syphilis, all kidney and prostatic symptoms are associated with depression and melancholia.	Restlessness, anxiety and weakness after micturition occur in the tubercular miasm.

Key Word	Psoric Urinary Symptoms	Sycotic Urinary Symptoms	Syphilitic Urinary Symptoms	Tubercular Urinary Symptoms
6. Flow	Psoric patients suffer from stress incontinence. The urine passes involuntarily and often frequently, when sneezing, coughing or laughing.	In sycosis, micturition is painful. There may be contraction of the urethra, and children will scream while urinating.	Most urinary complications are of sycotic origin, but when in combination with syphilis the result is diminished flow, and frequent desire for micturition with burning and irritation during the flow.	Colourless, profuse urination, thus diabetes is strongly tubercular.
	There may be burning and smarting while urinating resulting from acidic urine.	Scanty urination (psora is mainly responsible for scanty discharges/excretions), but during the rainy season polyuria is a characteristic of this miasm.	Irritation and burning of the parts, wherever the urine touches, indicates the acridity of this miasm.	The tubercular miasm is responsible for involuntary urination in children. Nocturnal enuresis in children should therefore undergo anti-tubercular treatment.
		In sycosis, there is a frequent desire to urinate before a thunderstorm.		
		Urinary cramps and painful spasms affecting the urethra and bladder may be present in sycosis.		
7. Kidneys	Fibrous changes in the kidneys are psoric in origin.	Sycotic patients suffer from renal calculi with pains, which are stitching and wandering in character.	Fibrous changes with destructive manifestations in kidneys.	In the tubercular miasm there may be recurrent, intermittent and periodic renal spasm with bleeding (haematuria), often noticed particularly during the new and full moon.
	Pain in kidney area, with inflammation of functional origin, nephritis, pyelitis, cystitis and urethritis.	Sycotic tumours of the kidneys or bladder are encapsulated and malignant.		

Key Word	Psoric Urinary Symptoms	Sycotic Urinary Symptoms	Syphilitic Urinary Symptoms	Tubercular Urinary Symptoms
8. Prostate	Psora has prostatitis (which incorporates a sycotic element) with oozing of prostatic fluid.	Enlargement of the prostate gland and complaints arising from it are sycotic.	Syphilitic patients suffer from carcinoma of the prostate with degenerative changes.	Prostate problems with bleeding per urethra are characteristic of the tubercular miasm.
9. Enuresis	In psora, enuresis occurs especially in children as a result of anxiety and fear (particularly a fear of going to school), or from other functional causes.	Enuresis is characterised by the patient waking up during urination due to some discomfort; and enuresis when habit is the only ascertainable cause (features of incoordination), are sycotic.	Syphilitic enuresis is characterised by a complete absence of the sense of realisation. The patient does not remember anything in the morning, lies on the wet bed and cannot be aroused.	The bed wetting of children soon after going to bed is tubercular with a sycotic element unless the patient wakes up during micturition, in which case the sycotic miasm predominates. Bed-wetting of chronic and recurrent character; which may also be periodic and intermittent is also tubercular as is nocturnal polyuria.
10. Urine	Psoric urine is generally dark but can also be yellowish or brownish.	A yellow colour represents sycosis.	Red, the colour of destruction, represents syphilis. Red coloured urine with streaks of pus is characteristic.	Albuminuria, and urine loaded with phosphate, sugar or protein are tubercular.
		Sycotic urine may have a fish-brine odour.		Tubercular urine is pale, colourless and copious. An offensive, musty and putrid, even carrion like odour may be present.
				Haematuria occurs during sleep.

MIASMATIC DIAGNOSIS:
<u>COMPARISON OF THE SEXUAL SYMPTOMS</u>

Key Word	Psoric Sexual Symptoms	Sycotic Sexual Symptoms	Syphilitic Sexual Symptoms	Tubercular Sexual Symptoms
1. Clinicals	Amenorrhoea.	In general, all varieties of sexual and pelvic disorders (including pelvic inflammatory diseases) come under the purview of sycosis.	Ulcerative and degenerative varieties of tumours are syphilitic.	All varieties of womb infections characterised by profuse bleeding are tubercular.
	Impotency and sterility from lack of sexual desire.	Uterine fibroids and polyps; ovarian tumours and malignancies where the tumour is encapsulated. Polycystic disease of the ovaries, and endometriosis are all sycotic.	Cervical and vulval erosion and ulceration.	Uterine and vaginal polyps with profuse bleeding.
		Leucorrhoea of fish brine odour.	Leucorrhoea, which is acrid, putrid and offensive.	DUB (dysfunctional uterine bleeding), which is characterised by profuse haemorrhage.
		Ectopic pregnancy.	Abortions and stillbirth.	Metastatic and haemorrhagic variety of cancers.
		Genital Warts.		Haemospermia (blood-stained seminal emissions).
		Sterility and infertility from hormonal imbalances.		

Key Word	Psoric Sexual Symptoms	Sycotic Sexual Symptoms	Syphilitic Sexual Symptoms	Tubercular Sexual Symptoms
2. Generals	Female: All functional menstrual disorders, especially amenorrhoea of functional origin.	Female: The sycotic patient experiences complications during labour, or delayed and painful labour, resulting in complications for the newborn child who suffers from various disorders.	Female: Recurrent abortions and stillbirth are syphilitic.	Female: In the tubercular miasm, weakness continues after menses, or during leucorrhoea and the patient may have sunken eyes and an anaemic appearance.
	Vaginal and uterine polypi are psora-syco-tubercular.	A mottled appearance of the mucous membrane of the endometrium is sycotic.	The syphilitic patient suffers from degenerative disorders and cervical dysplasia.	Exhaustive labour, with the exhaustion continuing after the birth and leaving the patient unable to nurse the child.
	During pregnancy the patient longs for peculiar things, which they no longer want when the desire is gratified and absolutely loath after gestation.	The uterus may be retroverted or retroflexed, with problems often occurring right after puberty.		Uterus retroverted or retroflexed as in sycosis, but in the tubercular miasm the condition is characterised by profuse uterine bleeding.
		Various disturbances from imbalance of the hormonal system, particularly around puberty and the menopause.		Climacteric flush (syco-tubercular).
	Male: The psoric mind may dwells on sexual matters (when this becomes truly excessive, a sycotic component must be present).	Male: Pain and swelling of the scrotum is sycotic. Hyper-sexuality.	Male: A perverted sexual appetite and perverted desires (e.g. with animals) characterises syphilis. Perverted sexuality.	Male: The tubercular male changes partners frequently and is never sexually satiated. Changeable sexuality.

Key Word	Psoric Sexual Symptoms	Sycotic Sexual Symptoms	Syphilitic Sexual Symptoms	Tubercular Sexual Symptoms
	Insufficient or deficient erection, even with the most voluptuous dreams or excitement. Hypo-sexuality (in organs) but restless mind. Dwindling, diminution or disappearance of one or both testicles is psoric.			
3. Sensation	Female: Dysmenorrhoea begins with puberty and is characterised by sharp pains.	Female: In sycosis, pruritus vulvae may occur with voluptuous itching; as a result of an imbalance in the acidic pH of the vaginal fluid.	Female: A burning, bursting sensation in the womb is a characteristic of syphilis.	Female: In the tubercular miasm the female patient often suffers from a sensation of great exhaustion.
4. Modalities	In psora we find aggravation from cold.	Sycosis finds aggravation from rest, a rainy or humid atmosphere and changes in the weather. Pruritus is aggravated by meat.	All symptoms of syphilis are aggravated at night, in summer and from warmth.	Tubercular manifestations are aggravated at night.
	Amelioration is from warmth in general and from natural discharges such as menstruation.	Amelioration is from unnatural discharges such as leucorrhoea (which are generally greenish/yellow). Amelioration by the return of suppressed normal discharges (e.g. menses).	Amelioration comes from any abnormal discharge such as leucorrhoea (this is also a sycotic manifestation).	Amelioration is from the open air.
5. Concomitants	Female: Psoric menstrual symptoms are associated with anxiety and mental restlessness.	Female: In sycosis, mental weakness is experienced during leucorrhoea.	Female: In syphilis we find depression from leucorrhoea or other uterine complications.	Female: Tubercular menstruation is accompanied by diarrhoea, weakness, vertigo, fainting and pallor of the face.

Key Word	Psoric Sexual Symptoms	Sycotic Sexual Symptoms	Syphilitic Sexual Symptoms	Tubercular Sexual Symptoms
			Melancholia and fears during menses.	Diarrhoea, fever, visual hallucinations of different colours, auditory hallucinations of different voices, anorexia, nausea, bitter vomiting and epistaxis during menses also typify the tubercular miasm. Hysterical manifestations may occur after menses. Extremities are cold and often menses can induce general anaemia in young women, and feelings of sadness, gloominess and anxiety. Menses is often accompanied by backache and headaches of all kinds. Leucorrhoea occurs with palpitations, faintness and loss of vitality in general but with a flushed face, vertigo, a dry, tickling, spasmodic cough and ringing in the ears.

Key Word	Psoric Sexual Symptoms	Sycotic Sexual Symptoms	Syphilitic Sexual Symptoms	Tubercular Sexual Symptoms
6. Discharges	Female: Psoric discharges are always bland and scanty. Scanty leucorrhoea. Offensive lochia with small clots. Nightly discharge of genital fluid, in women, with voluptuous dreams.	Female: Sycotic discharges are always profuse, can be yellowish or greenish/yellow. All discharges are of fish-brine smell, which is a characteristic.	Female: Syphilitic discharges are always acrid, putrid and offensive. Acrid and putrid leucorrhoea. Nightly discharge of genital fluid, in women, which is acrid and corrodes the part, wherever it touches.	Female: Tubercular discharges are always profuse and blood-tinged or haemorrhagic, can be associated with clots. Profuse bright red menses with clots. Even leucorrhoeal discharge can be mixed with blood or blood-tinged, can smell musty.
	Male: Nocturnal passing of semen may occur several times a week or even every night.	Male: Easy discharge of prostatic fluid with features of prostatitis during straining at stool or urination is characteristic.	Male: Azoospermia — dribbling of seminal fluid without the presence of sperm.	Male: Semen is emitted during defecation or micturition.
	Night pollution (scanty), easy ejaculation, impotency, and discharge of prostatic fluid during straining at stool or urination are psoric conditions.			Night pollution, a tendency to frequent masturbation, and uncontrolled, unrestrained sexual passion are characteristic of the tubercular miasm.
	Semen passes involuntarily during the daytime with little excitation, and often without erection.			Spermatorrhoea occurs at nightfall and during sleep without dreams.

Key Word	Psoric Sexual Symptoms	Sycotic Sexual Symptoms	Syphilitic Sexual Symptoms	Tubercular Sexual Symptoms
7. Sexual Desire	Female: In psora we find a lack of sexual desire (in both sexes).	Female: In sycosis, sexual desire is increased, resulting in various sexual fantasies, voluptuous desires and a nymphomaniac state.	Female: Syphilitic sexual desires are perverted and can include sexual violence, sadism etc.	Female: Unrestrained, uncontrolled passions including masturbation (in both sexes), and over-indulgence in sex, to the point of perversion, which ultimately leads to exhaustion and becomes detrimental to the health.
	Male: In psora, the erection may be incomplete, short or lacking.	Male: Hyper-sexuality is evident in the sycotic miasm.	Male: In the syphilitic male, sexual cravings are perverted or completely destroyed.	Male: In the tubercular miasm, masturbation is followed by the loss of all enthusiasm leading to depression followed by weakness of memory.
8. Fertility	Female: In psora there may be sterility or impotence without any organic defect in the sexual parts. There are general or sexual weaknesses and deficient desire or orgasm.	Female: Sycosis being the miasm of incoordination results in the incapability to conceive due to various factors including hormonal imbalances. In sycosis, sterility and infertility result from pelvic inflammatory diseases and other conditions such as endometriosis.	Female: Possible failure to discharge the ovum at ovulation resulting in infertility is a syphilitic condition.	Female: In the tubercular miasm, infertility results from prolonged menstrual bleeding.
	Male: The psoric male may suffer from oligospermia (low sperm count).		Male: The syphilitic male suffers from azoospermia (complete absence of spermatozoa), which results in infertility.	

Key Word	Psoric Sexual Symptoms	Sycotic Sexual Symptoms	Syphilitic Sexual Symptoms	Tubercular Sexual Symptoms
9. Menstruation	Scanty (as psora reflects 'hypo'), watery menses.	Sycosis has various menstrual disorders including itching pudenda, pruritus vulvae, mastodynia (breast pain) and polyuria during menses.	In syphilis there is profuse menstrual flow, which is acrid and offensive, and the menstrual blood has a metallic odour.	In the tubercular miasm, menses is exhaustive and prolonged with copious, bright red blood often containing lots of clots.
	In psora, the menses are slow in setting in after puberty and may appear one or more times and then cease for several months or even for a year before returning.	Sycotic menses has the odour of fish-brine, and the stain of the menstrual blood is difficult to wash off.	Irregular periods are syphilitic, with irregularity in both quantity and frequency.	Tubercular menses often appear too soon, perhaps every 2-3 weeks. They may or may not be painful, but are always exhausting. The patient feels poorly a week before menstruation starts.
	Retarded, protracted menses, and retarded menses of short duration are characteristic of psora.	Menstrual pains are spasmodic, extremely sharp and colicky, often coming in paroxysms. The flow may come only with the pains.	Depression and fears during menses are syphilitic.	Flow can also be pale but long lasting, often resulting in anaemia.
	Foetid blood.	Sycotic menses are abundant (tubercular component is present too) and painful.	Syphilitic menses are characterised by bone pains and lumbago.	Tuberculars have profuse and/ or long lasting menstrual bleeding.

Key Word	Psoric Sexual Symptoms	Sycotic Sexual Symptoms	Syphilitic Sexual Symptoms	Tubercular Sexual Symptoms
	Dysmenorrhoea may occur at puberty or at the climacteric, and pains are sharp but never colicky.	Menstrual flow is acrid (the acridity component is rendered by syphilis), excoriating and biting, and there may be burning of the pudendum. The discharge is clotted, stringy (stringiness is generally syphilitic, but can be sycotic when it is characterised by the cause, i.e. an incoordination) and yellowish.		Dysmenorrhoea is exhaustive, draining the patient totally.
10. Coition	Female: Psora has weakness of the sexual organs as a result of prolonged suffering from exhaustive diseases.	Female: In sycosis there is hyper-excitation and frequent sexual arousal.	Female: In syphilis, an inability to perform coitus, and decreased sexual power can be associated with a burning, acrid, sore feeling in the vagina.	Female: The tubercular patient suffers from painful coitus due to polyps in the vulva and vagina.
	Male: Premature ejaculation is characteristic of psoric males.	Male: In sycosis, erections are frequent and strong.	Male: In syphilis, erections are troublesome, strong and painful and may occur without any sexual desire.	Male: The tubercular male suffers from painful erections and coitus, but is still prone to strong sexual indulgence.

MIASMATIC DIAGNOSIS:
COMPARISON OF THE DERMATOLOGICAL SYMPTOMS

Key Word	Psoric Skin	Sycotic Skin	Syphilitic Skin	Tubercular Skin
1. Clinicals	Psora has eczema and eruptions of all kinds in which dryness predominates.	The sycotic patient is subject to warts, veruccas, moles, condylomatas, skin tags, dermoid cysts, fibromas and lipomas. Genital warts may appear in both sexes.	Ulcers and abscesses on different parts of the skin are syphilitic.	Any skin condition characterised by recurrence, periodicity, alternation or haemorrhage. Tubercular conditions are obstinate and difficult to eradicate.
	Pimples with dryness and scurfy scales.	Vesicular eruptions are generally sycotic.	Necrosis, gangrene and bedsores.	Allergic skin manifestations; urticaria.
	Dandruff with bran-like scales.	Herpes of all types.	Deep cracks and fissures in the skin (mainly the palms and soles).	Herpes, which is extremely recurrent and may be periodic.
	Nettle rash is of psoric origin but can only manifest as a combination of two miasms, mainly psora-tubercular (as allergies are tubercular).	Hyperpigmentation of the skin, and melanomas are sycotic.	Depigmentation (destruction of pigmentation) of the skin.	Haemangiomas.
		Keloids, corns with thickening of the skin and post-operative scar tumours.	Stitch abscesses.	Recurrent pustular eczemas.
		Radiation hazards resulting in cauliflower-like tumours.	Skin cancer characterised by ulceration and necrosis is syphilitic.	Venous thrombosis and varicose veins with red flushing.

Key Word	Psoric Skin	Sycotic Skin	Syphilitic Skin	Tubercular Skin
		Molluscum contagiosum (syco-psoric).	Burns and scalds with degenerative ulceration.	Petechial haemorrhage, ecchymosis and purpura are tubercular.
		The consequences of vaccinosis.		Ulcerations with haemorrhage.
2. General	Ringworm (more tuberculo-psoric or tuberculo-sycotic, according to the cause and manifestations), itch and eczema are not of psora but the results of psora.	In sycosis, we find disturbed pigment metabolism, resulting in hyper-pigmentation in patches or diffused in different parts.	Ulcerative and degenerative skin conditions are syphilitic.	The tubercular miasm has skin diseases of threatening or destructive natures.
	Tendency of recurrent skin diseases is psoric in origin but psora-tubercular in manifestation (as recurrence is tubercular).	Hypertrophied conditions of the skin are sycotic.	Syphilis has an ulcerous tendency, particularly towards virulent types of open ulcers.	The areas affected tend to be those which are subjected to much use. Eruptions therefore are evident around the fingers and lips, and in or around the mouth.
	In psora, scratching eruptions are followed by dry scales.	Circumscribed or circular patches of hyper-pigmentation in different areas of the skin.	Eruptions, which are slow to heal, are syphilo-psoric.	The tubercular miasm encompasses the state where there is a presence of ringworm or where there has been a past history of the suppression of ringworm.
	Eczemas and eruptions are papular and associated with itching.	Fish scale eruptions can be syco-psoric or tri-miasmatic, combining the dryness of psora, the thickened skin of sycosis and the squamous character of syphilis.	Ulcerated skin with pus and blood represents syphilis.	Recurrent and obstinate boils with profuse pus.

Key Word	Psoric Skin	Sycotic Skin	Syphilitic Skin	Tubercular Skin
	Voluptuous tickling and itching, which is only temporarily relieved by rubbing and scratching.	Painful skin eruptions which are localised and/or in circumscribed spots.		Skin conditions associated with glandular involvement are tubercular.
	Psoric skin diseases are devoid of suppuration and apt to be dry.	Vesicular eruptions which do not heal quickly and urine-coloured patches are sycotic.		
3. Sensation	Sensation of burning.		Syphilitic skin is not itchy but there can be sensations of rawness and soreness.	In the tubercular miasm, a sensation of exhaustion is present with skin diseases.
	Unhealthy skin with itching and burning represents psora.			
	Pruritus is always a manifestation of psora.	Pruritis (is of psoric origin) but manifests in sycosis in the anus, nose and sexual organs with thickening of the skin.		
4. Modalities	In psora, itching often occurs late in the evening before midnight and is most unbearable.	Sycotic skin eruptions are aggravated by the consumption of meat; in humid and rainy weather, and from changes in the weather generally.	All symptoms of syphilis are aggravated at night, in summer, from the warmth of the bed and from warmth in general.	Tubercular skin diseases are aggravated at night, by touch and pressure generally, while thinking of complaints, after undressing, from milk, greasy and oily foods, from the warmth of the bed (syphilitic component), and after itching.
	Psoric skin complaints are aggravated by cold, in winter, and from undressing.			

Key Word	Psoric Skin	Sycotic Skin	Syphilitic Skin	Tubercular Skin
	Amelioration is from natural discharges such as sweat.	In sycosis there is amelioration in dry weather.	Amelioration of the syphilitic miasm comes with any abnormal discharge.	Amelioration is from the open air, and dry weather.
	Relief also comes from the reappearance of suppressed skin eruptions.	When warts or fibrous growths reappear, the sycotic patient feels relieved.		
		Painful skin eruptions are better by pressure.		
oncomitants	In psora, when skin diseases are suppressed the mind is directly affected, resulting in anxiety, apprehension, and fear of incurable diseases.	Suppression of sycotic skin diseases affects first the nerve centres of the body and then the heart, liver and reproductive system. Hyperaesthesia, cardiac incoordinations including dropsy; hepatomegaly and various pelvic inflammatory disorders including endometriosis may result.	Leprosy in which liquefaction has already started is tubercular but with syphilis predominating.	When tubercular skin is suppressed, it affects the inner tissues causing destructive and ulcerous tendencies, and the deeper tissues causing debilitated tubercular states such as fatigue syndromes.
		Suppression of ringworm can result in rheumatism, chronic headaches, stomach complaints and chronic bronchitis.	When syphilitic skin is suppressed the intellect is affected, causing dullness, depression and a lack of enthusiasm.	
pearance	Psoric skin appears dirty, dry and harsh and becomes more dry with washing. The skin cannot endure water and often has an unwashed, unhealthy, dingy look.	Small, reddish, flat vesicular eruptions which are slow to heal (in slow healing the syphilitic miasmatic taint must also be present) and recur during the menstrual period are sycotic.	Threatening (ulcerative and destructive) appearance.	Tubercular skin conditions are angry looking and often accompanied by oozing of blood.

Key Word	Psoric Skin	Sycotic Skin	Syphilitic Skin	Tubercular Skin
	Cracks on the hands and feet with extreme dryness.	Warty excrescences, which appear after vaccinations.	Ulcerating moles with hairy tufts are syphilitic.	Skin lesions are red and haemorrhagic in appearance.
		Red pinhead type moles and other moles, warts, wine coloured patches (multi-miasmatic with underlying sycosis), urine coloured patches and other manifestations of unnaturally thickened skin.	Syphilitic eruptions are found around the joints and flexures of the body and are arranged in circular groupings (in all circular and circumscribed manifestations sycosis is also present), rings or segments of circles.	
		Spider web, red capillaries over the centre of the malar bone.	Copper or raw ham coloured eruptions.	
		Acne, which is red in appearance (in red appearance the tubercular miasm is also present), angry looking, papular or vesicular eruptions around the time of the menstrual period, which are isolated and painful.	Putridity and offensiveness of all discharges with ugly looking ulcers, which have a cadaverous base.	
		Sycotic skin looks oily and the tip of the nose appears red. There may be stubby, dead, broken hair in the beard, which falls out due to skin eruptions.		

Key Word	Psoric Skin	Sycotic Skin	Syphilitic Skin	Tubercular Skin
7. Colour	Psoric eruptions are not noticeable by their colour but by the roughness of the skin.	Sycosis has a disturbed pigment metabolism producing both hyper and depigmentation, which occurs in patches or is diffused in different parts.	In syphilis, there are copper coloured eruptions, which do not heal fast, but turn to ulceration. The discomfort is aggravated at night and by the warmth of the bed.	Tubercular skin is pale with a bluish tint showing signs of venous stagnation.
				Varicose veins have a red flushed appearance.
				Freckles are quite significant especially in fine, transparent, smooth-skinned people.
8. Eruptions	Itching without pus or discharge is characteristic of psora.	Exfoliating eczemas are sycotic.	Syphilis has a tendency to develop open ulcers of virulent type. All eruptions are patchy.	Eczema, and ringworm, a history of ringworm and suppression of ringworm are tubercular.
	Warts (syco-psoric) on face, arms and hands, with dryness.	Fish scale eruptions are tri-miasmatic but mainly sycotic in manifestation due to the thickening of the skin and the exfoliative tendency.	Ulcers and putrefaction of all tissues devoid of pain and itching.	Urticaria and herpes (allergic and recurrent varieties e.g. recurrent herpes genitalis). If eruptions are pustular or vesicular the suppuration (coming from the syphilitic component) is marked.
	Psoriasis has been called "the marriage of all the miasms but its characteristics are predominantly psoric and sycotic". (Dr. Roberts).	Herpes (including herpes zoster and genitalis), erysipelas, all sorts of warts and excrescences, barber's itch and other scaly and patchy skin eruptions, which occur in circumscribed spots.	All sorts of ulcers, carbuncles and boils, which do not heal fast (slow to heal is psora-syphilitic) and are characterised by the discharge of offensive and spreading fluid and pus are syphilitic.	Painful eruptions in the vagina during pregnancy are characteristic of a prominent tubercular miasm.

Key Word	Psoric Skin	Sycotic Skin	Syphilitic Skin	Tubercular Skin
	Crusts, which are thin, light, fine and small, are present in psora.	Post-operative scar tumours and proliferation of the stitch line after an operation are sycotic.	Stitch abscesses, malignant dyscrasias; gangrenes of the skin and dry gangrene are all syphilitic manifestations.	The formation of pus after insect or fly bites or the slightest injury, which does not heal fast is tubercular.
	Small, sensitive, painful, non-suppurating boils, which may shed scurfy scales.	All sorts of facial skin diseases that may be contracted at the barber's, such as tinea barbae and tinea vesicular, but excluding tinea favosa.	All skin conditions characterised by putridity and offensiveness of discharges.	Recurrent stitch abscesses after an operation or scarring after ulcers are generally associated with bleeding in the tubercular miasm. Recurrent and obstinate boils with profuse pus and fever, heal with difficulty.
		Abnormal growths (a combination of sycosis with the tubercular miasm).	Crusts are always thick (in thickening of the crust, sycosis also plays a role; as thickening is a proliferation or excess deposition) and heavy.	Abnormal growths (with clearness of the skin).
9. Sweat	Scanty, sour smelling sweat, especially on forehead and during sleep is psoric.	In sycosis, sweat appears on the forehead during sleep. The skin has an oily appearance and perspiration is thick and copious.	Syphilitic sweat is offensive and aggravates all complaints.	In the tubercular miasm there is offensive foot or axillary sweat which when suppressed may induce lung trouble or some other severe disease.
10. Parasites	Animal parasites with tickling in the skin and voluptuous itching (voluptuousness is an excessive component rendered by sycosis) are psoric.	Parasitic infestation with thickening of the skin is sycotic.	Parasitic infestation with ulceration of the skin is syphilitic.	Animal parasitic infestations with tickling and bleeding are tubercular.

MIASMATIC DIAGNOSIS:
<u>COMPARISON OF THE NAIL SYMPTOMS</u>

Key Word	Psoric Nails	Sycotic Nails	Syphilitic Nails	Tubercular Nails
1. Nails	Psoric nails have a dry, harsh appearance.	Sycotic nails are thick as a result of hyper or excess deposition of tissue.	Syphilitic nails are thin (as a result of destruction of the cells) and bend and tear easily.	The tubercular miasm has frequent and recurrent brittle nails, which often drop off and then grow again.
	On pressing the tip of the nail, the nail beds present an anaemic appearance.	Ridges or ribs, which can be longitudinal or horizontal, are visible on the nails.	Pitted nails with indentations, or longitudinal or transverse indentations, like grooves or channels in the nails.	Nails with various stains, glossy nails with white specks and scalloped edges, and spotted nails are all tubercular. On pressing the tip of the nail, there occurs red flushing in the nail bed.
		Wavy, corrugated nails with protuberance or bumps are sycotic.	Syphilitic nails have brittle edges, which bend easily.	Asymmetrical nails, which come out easily are tubercular.
		Dome-shaped nails with a convex appearance.	Spoon-shaped; concave nails (the reverse of sycosis).	The natural convexity is often reversed.
		Irregular (feature of incoordination) shaped nails with irregular but thick edges.	Whitlows and panaritium, with pus points at the end or corners of the nails.	Irregular nails, which break and split easily.
		Stitching pains may occur in the nail beds.		Formation of pus at the junction of the nail and flesh, with many hang nails.

MIASMATIC DIAGNOSIS:
<u>COMPARISON OF THE EXTREMITY SYMPTOMS</u>

Key Word	Psoric Extremities	Sycotic Extremities	Syphilitic Extremities	Tubercular Extremities
1. Clinicals	Various types of rheumatism, especially of a functional and inflammatory nature; osteitis, osteomyelitis (the initial stage without bone destruction. When the destruction starts, the condition becomes syphilitic); periostitis.	Osteoporosis is syco-syphilitic (the hormonal imbalance is given by sycosis and bone porosis or destruction is afforded by syphilis).	Bone pains, delayed ossification and fragility of the bones; caries and necrosis of the bones and spine are syphilitic.	Rickets are syphilo-tubercular.
	Leg cramps.	Rheumatism, gout and osteoarthritis.	Osteomyelitis with bone destruction and formation of sequestrum.	Nodular growths of glandular origin.
		All joint pains of the small and larger joints are sycotic.	Malignancy of the bones, bone metastasis and sarcoma.	Weakness of the ankle joints.
		Arthritic deformans; tophi and deposits in the joints.	Ulcers and gangrenous inflammations.	Offensive and sweaty palms and soles.
		Oedematous swelling of the extremities.	Paralysis characterised by muscle wasting and degenerative changes (when incoordination and malfunctioning are evident, paralysis is sycotic).	
2. Generals	The extremity pains of psora are generally neuralgic in type.	Incoordination, which may be anatomical or functional, is characteristic of sycosis.	Syphilis shows an extremely irregular development of symptoms.	Pupura and haemorrhagic manifestations are characteristic of the tubercular miasm.

Key Word	Psoric Extremities	Sycotic Extremities	Syphilitic Extremities	Tubercular Extremities
	Sore, bruised and pressive pains are psoric.	The sycotic diathesis is rheumatic and gouty.	Pain in the long bones is syphilitic.	Delayed milestones.
		Sycosis is silent or even surreptitious in its manifestations.		Weakness of the ankle joints is a sure indication of the presence of syphilo-psora, i.e. the tubercular miasm.
		Joints and connective tissues are affected.		
3. Sensation	Sensations of dryness, heat and burning of the hands and feet with sweating of the palms and soles are characteristic of psora.	Rheumatism, numbness and paralytic weakness of the extremities are sycotic.	Burning, bursting and tearing sensations are syphilitic.	Cramps in the lower extremities, legs, feet and toes are tubercular but also found in psora.
	Numbness with tingling sensations; feeling as if parts are going to sleep, which occurs when pressure is brought to bear on the part, when lying lightly on the part or when sitting cross-legged.	Joint pains; stitching, pulsating, shooting, tearing and wandering pains are sycotic. Shooting, and tearing pains may occur in the muscles as well as the joints. Stiffness, soreness, lameness are also characteristic of sycosis.		
	Pricking and tingling in the extremities due to 'hypo' or poor circulation, with coldness of the extremities.	Gouty concretions due to rheumatic affection, with pain in the joints or periosteum with inflammatory deposits.		
	Leg cramps.	Proliferative variety of inflammation or growth of any tissues.		
	Constant chilliness.			

Key Word	Psoric Extremities	Sycotic Extremities	Syphilitic Extremities	Tubercular Extremities
4. Modalities	Psoric aggravation occurs in winter. The patient requires warmth both externally and internally.	Pains are worse at the approach of a storm or during a thunderstorm (generally thunderstorm aggravations are predominantly tubercular or syphilo-tubercular; but can also be present in sycosis due to incoordination), from damp humid atmosphere and rainy weather.	Syphilitic pains are worse at night or at the approach of night, and there is general aggravation from sunset to sunrise. The seaside, sea voyages, thunderstorms, summer and warmth, and extremes of temperature also aggravate.	In the tubercular miasm, aggravation comes at night and from thunderstorms.
	Aggravation also occurs between sunrise and sunset, from cold and from standing.	Rheumatic pains are worse from cold and damp, rest, changes in the weather and from meat.	Acute rheumatic pain, osteomyelitis and ulcerous inflammation in the bone marrow with its accompanying pains, are aggravated at night and during stormy weather and changes in the weather.	Milk, fruits, and greasy and oily foods aggravate.
		Stooping, bending and beginning to move also aggravate sycotic conditions.	Movement, perspiration and the warmth of the bed cause aggravation in syphilis.	Tubercular patients cannot tolerate any pressure to the chest and feel worse in a closed room.
			Syphilitic and tubercular pains are similar in character and times of aggravation.	
	Psoric amelioration is evident in the summer, from heat, and by natural discharges such as urine, sweat, menstruation etc. Physiological eliminative processes like diarrhoea, also ameliorate.	Better by moving, from slow motion, stretching and rubbing, pressure, by lying on the stomach and in dry weather.	In syphilis, there is amelioration from sunrise to sunset, in lukewarm climates and during the winter cold. Changes in position also ameliorate.	Neuralgic pains are better by quiet, rest and warmth. Aggravated from motion.

Key Word	Psoric Extremities	Sycotic Extremities	Syphilitic Extremities	Tubercular Extremities
	Psoric conditions are also ameliorated by hot application, scratching, crying and eating, and the appearance of suppressed skin eruptions.	Sycotic conditions are ameliorated by unnatural discharges (which are generally greenish-yellow), and by unnatural elimination through the mucus surfaces, such as leucorrhoea, nasal discharge etc. Physiological eliminations however do not ameliorate.	Syphilitic conditions are better for any abnormal discharges such as leucorrhoea and coryza and from the discharge of pus when old ulcers break open.	Amelioration is from dry weather, open air, and in the daytime.
		The return of suppressed normal discharges such as menses ameliorate, as do the appearance of warts and fibrous growths.		Temporary amelioration comes from offensive foot or axillary sweat which when suppressed induces lung trouble.
		Ameliorated in general from the return or breaking open of old ulcers and old sores, and markedly ameliorated by the return of acute gonorrhoeal manifestations.		Amelioration from nosebleeds is characte tubercular miasm.
5. Character	In psora there is twitching of the muscles during sleep.	The slightest physical exertion fatigues the sycotic patient.	Aching pains in the bones of the limbs and in the joints are syphilitic.	The tubercular patient is unable to tolerate exertion and lack of exercise leads to flabbiness.
	Various types of rheumatism, especially of functional inflammatory nature without gross structural changes; curvature of the bones, osteitis and osteomyelitis are characteristic of psora.	Easy spraining of the joints while walking; joints and connective tissues which are easily affected, are sycotic.	In syphilis, the ankle joint is weak and the patient stumbles and falls easily.	

Key Word	Psoric Extremities	Sycotic Extremities	Syphilitic Extremities	Tubercular Extremities
		Stiffness, soreness and lameness are characteristic of sycosis, and gouty diatheses have a sycotic base.	The syphilitic stigmata may affect the bony structures causing destructive changes (e.g. osteomalacia).	Profuse perspiration occurs on the palms of the hands and the soles of the feet.
			Burning, bursting and tearing pains are syphilitic, and shooting or lancinating pains may occur in the periosteum or long bones.	Offensive, sweaty palms and soles. Cold, damp, soft and flabby hands, and a coldness of the hands and feet of which the patient is not always conscious.
				Tubercular patients have weak wrist and ankle joints and difficulty holding on to objects. They drop things easily, are clumsy in getting about and stumble over the tiniest things.
6. Appearance	The psoric patient suffers from prominent varicose veins in the lower part of the body.	Sycosis has anatomical abnormalities such as six fingers.	The syphilitic patient may be subject to various deformities and atrophy of various organs.	Nodular growths are tubercular.
		Local or generalised oedema or anasarca is characteristic in sycosis.	A marasmic appearance is basically syphilitic because the syphilitic stigma destroys the power of the body to assimilate proper materials from food.	Tubercular patients often have distinctive fingers, which may be either equal and long with blunt or club-shaped tips which do not appear converged, or long and irregularly arranged. The hands are thin, soft and flabby and can easily be compressed. They are also usually very moist, often cold and damp, and perspire profusely.

Key Word	Psoric Extremities	Sycotic Extremities	Syphilitic Extremities	Tubercular Extremities
7. Function	In psora, the patient can walk well and finds it difficult to stand still.	Sycosis infiltrates and corrodes (syphilo-sycosis) by its discharges and smells of fish brine.	Syphilis has paralytic weaknesses caused by destruction or severe impairment of the functions of the nerves and muscles.	Rickets may occur in the tubercular miasm causing soft and curved bones.
		In sycosis, the red blood corpuscles are destroyed through imperfect oxidisation of food. This can lead to anaemic conditions, which may be evidenced by a lack of stamina in the muscles and a pallid, drawn, puffy appearance.		Drop wrists, a weakness and loss of power in the tendons around the joints and tendons and ligaments which sprain easily. The ankles turn easily from the slightest misstep and activities such as playing the piano and typing cause exhaustion and swelling of the fingers and wrist joints.
		Chronic or long-continued inflammation is characteristic especially in the joints.		There is a general lack of energy and a lack of strength in the bones.
		The sycotic miasm is devoid of power. The joints are easily sprained even while walking and there is numbness of the extremities.		The feet are cold and damp and perspire profusely, a fact of which the patient is unaware.
				The slightest physical exertion fatigues the tubercular patient and there is a great sense of exhaustion. As the sun ascends, their strength revives, and as it descends they lose it again. Tiredness comes on at night even after a sleep.

Key Word	Psoric Sleep	Sycotic Sleep	Syphilitic Sleep	Tubercular Sleep
1. Character of sleep and dream	Sleep: Psoric sleep is unrefreshing with fearful dreams and dreams of anxiety. There is weariness on awakening.	Sleep: The sycotic patient sleeps for a short time, wakes, then returns to sleep again.	Sleep: Rolling the head from side to side during sleep is characteristic of syphilis.	Sleep: The tubercular patient screams out during sleep.
	Twitching of muscles during sleep.	Restless sleep is characteristic of sycosis.		Sleep is accompanied by a sensation of great exhaustion.
	Loud talking and screaming during sleep.			
	Gnashing of teeth during sleep and expulsion of round worms.			
	Somnambulism occurs in psora and there is sleeplessness during the day.			
	Dreams: As soon as the psoric patient closes their eyes, fearful images and distorted faces appear.	Dreams: The sycotic patient has sexual dreams with fantasies.	Dreams: Sexual dreams with perversions and suicidal dreams are syphilitic.	Dreams: The tubercular patient dreams of travelling.
	Dreams are vivid (as if the patient were awake); sad, frightful, anxious and lascivious.		The syphilitic patient dreams of violence; destruction, death and dead bodies, and generally gloomy forebodings.	

Key Word	Psoric Sleep	Sycotic Sleep	Syphilitic Sleep	Tubercular Sleep
2. Modalities	Psoric complaints are aggravated during sleep.	In sycosis, sleep is restless in damp, humid weather and during thunderstorms.	Syphilitic sleep is disturbed at the seaside, during the summer, at night and from sweat. Amelioration comes from a change of position.	Tubercular sleep is disturbed in enclosed, stuffy rooms.
3. Concomitants	Psoric sleeplessness is experienced due to an abundance of ideas. Sweating, especially on the head, snoring, salivation, grinding of the teeth, unconsciousness, and passing of stool and urine during sleep are all characteristic of psora.	In sycosis, sleeplessness occurs due to mental and physical disquiet.	The syphilitic patient is sleepless because of tormenting ideas. Sleep is unrefreshing and accompanied by depression and melancholia.	Unrefreshing sleep with great exhaustion is tubercular.

MIASMATIC DIAGNOSIS:
COMPARISON OF MODALITY SYMPTOMS

Key Word	Psoric Modalities	Sycotic Modalities	Syphilitic Modalities	Tubercular Modalities
1. Aggravation	Psora has aggravation in winter and during sleep.	Sycotic aggravation is from rest, damp cold, moist cold, the rainy season, humid atmosphere, from changes in the weather, during thunderstorms and from heat.	In syphilis there is aggravation from sunset to sunrise, from natural discharges such as perspiration, from extremes of temperature, at the seaside and from sea voyages, from thunderstorms, movement, during the summer, from warmth and from the warmth of the bed.	Worse during thunderstorm (like sycosis and syphilis), and at night.
	Wants warmth both internally and externally (aggravation from cold).	Pains in the joints are worse during cold, damp weather.		The tubercular patient cannot tolerate any pressure in the chest.
	Psora is associated with mental restlessness and anxiety. The patient cannot stand still and must walk instead of standing.	The sycotic patient is like a barometer — he has pains when it rains, and when the atmosphere is filled with moisture he suffers.		In the tubercular miasm there is aggravation from milk, fruits, greasy and oily foods and in closed rooms.
2. Amelioration	Sunrise to sunset.	The sycotic patient gains amelioration from motion, during winter, in a dry atmosphere and from any unnatural discharge such as leucorrhoea or catarrh. Natural eliminations do not ameliorate.	Syphilitic amelioration occurs from sunrise to sunset, from a change of position, in lukewarm climates, during winter, from cold and from any abnormal discharge such as leucorrhoea.	In the tubercular miasm, there is amelioration in dry weather, open air and during the daytime.

Key Word	Psoric Modalities	Sycotic Modalities	Syphilitic Modalities	Tubercular Modalities
	In summer, by heat or warmth in general, and from hot applications.	Mental conditions may be much ameliorated when warts or fibrous growths appear, and there is a general amelioration from the return or breaking open of old ulcers and sores. There is also a marked amelioration from the return of acute gonorrhoeal manifestations.	Conditions improve through the discharge of pus (better if old ulcer opens up).	Temporary amelioration is by offensive foot or axillary sweat, which when suppressed, induces lung conditions.
	The psoric patient has a desire to lie down day and night for amelioration of his troubles.	Joint pains are ameliorated in the morning or by stretching, in dry weather and by slow motion.		Amelioration by epistaxis is characteristic of the tubercular miasm.
	Amelioration from natural discharges such as urine and menses, and better through physiological eliminative processes such as perspiration.	Amelioration from lying on stomach, pressure, or return of suppressed normal discharge (e.g. menses).		
3. Process	Psora develops physical irritation, i.e. itch.	Sycosis develops catarrhal discharges.	Syphilis produces open ulcers.	The tubercular miasm produces haemorrhages.

MIASMATIC DIAGNOSIS:
COMPARISON OF CHARACTERISTICS: A SYNOPSIS

Key Word	Psora Sensitising Miasm	Sycosis Miasm of Incoordination	Syphilis Degenerating Miasm	Tubercular Responsive, Reactive Miasm
1. General Manifestations	i) Psora develops itch.	i) Sycosis develops catarrhal discharges.	i) The syphilitic miasm has virulent open ulcers.	i) The tubercular miasm has haemorrhages.
	ii) Unhealthy skin with burning and itching represents psora.	ii) Oily skin with thickly oozing and copious perspiration, represents sycosis.	ii) Ulcerated skin with pus and blood represents syphilis.	ii) Oily skin with coldness represents the tubercular miasm.
	iii) All 'hypos' are mainly psoric.	iii) 'Hypers' are sycotic.	iii) 'Dyses' are syphilitic.	iii) Allergies are tubercular.
	iv) Hypoplasia is psoric.	iv) Hyperplasia is sycotic.	iv) Dysplasia is syphilitic.	iv) Alternation of 'hypo' and dysplasia is tubercular.
	v) Atrophy, ataxia, anaemia and anoxaemia are psoric.	v) Hypertrophy is sycotic.	v) Dystrophy is syphilitic.	v) Dystrophy with haemorrhage is tubercular.
	vi) Hypotension is psoric.	vi) Hypertension is sycotic.	vi) Irregular, arrhythmic pulse is syphilitic.	vi) Intermittent pulse is tubercular.
	vii) Lack, scanty, less and absence denote psora.	vii) Exaggeration or excess denotes sycosis.	vii) Destruction and degeneration denotes syphilis.	vii) Alternation and periodicity is tubercular.
	viii) Weakness is psoric.	viii) Restlessness (especially physical) is sycotic.	viii) Destructiveness is syphilitic.	viii) Changeableness is tubercular.

Key Word	Psora Sensitising Miasm	Sycosis Miasm of Incoordination	Syphilis Degenerating Miasm	Tubercular Responsive, Reactive Miasm
	ix) An inhibitory quality is psoric in nature.	ix) An expressive quality is characteristic of sycosis.	ix) Melancholic, depressive and suicidal tendencies are syphilitic in nature.	ix) A dissatisfied quality is tubercular in nature.
	x) Dryness of membranes denotes psora.	x) Augmented secretion denotes sycosis.	x) Ulceration denotes syphilis.	x) Haemorrhages and allergies denote the tubercular miasm.
	xi) Psora does not assimilate well.	xi) Sycotics are over nourished.	xi) Syphilitics has disorganised digestion.	xi) Tubercular patients crave the things which make them sick.
	xii) The secretions of psora are serous.	xii) Sycotic secretions are purulent.	xii) The secretions of syphilis are sticky, acrid and putrid.	xii) Tubercular secretions are haemorrhagic.
2. General Nature of the Miasm	Hyper-sensitivity (basically psora is 'hypo' in expression which gives rise to hypo-immunity, in turn resulting in hyper-susceptibility which manifests as an exalted sensitivity to the external environment and allergens). Itching, irritation and burning lead towards congestion and inflammation with only functional changes. The capacity to produce hyper-sensitivity, i.e. the sensitising property of psora is its basic nature.	Sycosis produces incoordination everywhere resulting in over production, growth, and infiltration in the form of warts, condylomata, tumours, fibrous tissues etc.	Syphilis produces destructive disorder everywhere, which manifests as perversion, suppuration, ulceration and fissures.	The tubercular miasm produces changing symptomatology, confusing vague symptomatology (e.g. dyspepsia, weakness, wasting, fever), and conditions which are variable, shifting in location, changing in outlook, alternating in state, and contradictory.
3. Key Words & Expressions	Hypo-immunity.	Hyper — mental and physical.	Destruction — physical and mental.	Dissatisfaction.

Key Word	Psora Sensitising Miasm	Sycosis Miasm of Incoordination	Syphilis Degenerating Miasm	Tubercular Responsive, Reactive Miasm
	Anxiety and apprehension.	Hypertrophy — growths and incoordinations.	Degeneration.	Alternation, changeability, and migratory conditions.
	Alertness.		Necrosis and ulceration.	Periodic, recurrent and allergic.
	Fears.		Putridity and acridity.	Vague manifestations.
	Irritation — mental and physical.		'Dyses'	Craves the things which make them sick.
	Sensitivity.		Irregular and arrhythmic.	
4. Diathesis	i) Eruptive.	i) Rheumatic and gouty.	i) Suppurative or ulcerative.	i) Scrofulous.
		ii) Lithic and uric acid.		ii) Haemorrhagic.
		iii) Proliferative.		iii) Allergic.
5. Organs & Tissues Affected	Ectodermal tissues. Nervous system, endocrine system, blood vessels, liver and skin.	Entodermal tissues — soft tissues. Attacks internal organs, the blood (producing anaemias), and the pelvis and sexual organs.	Mesodermal tissues and bones, and the glandular tissues particularly the lymphatics.	Glandular tissue. The patient is poor in bone, flesh and blood.
6. Nature of Diseases	i) Deficiency disorders.	i) Deposition and/or proliferation of cells/tissues.	i) Destructive, degenerative disorders, deformities and fragility.	i) Depletion.
				ii) Drainage and wasting.
				iii) Alternating disorders.

Key Word	Psora Sensitising Miasm	Sycosis Miasm of Incoordination	Syphilis Degenerating Miasm	Tubercular Responsive, Reactive Miasm
7. Pace of Action	i) Hyperactive.	i) Extremely slow, insidious.	i) Usually midway in pace, i.e. moderate. Though sometimes may be rapid or insidious.	i) Depends according to preponderance of psoric or syphilitic miasm.
	ii) Dramatic development of symptoms.	ii) Silent or even surreptitious in its manifestations.	ii) Irregular/arrhythmic pace.	
			iii) Generally more overt in its manifestations.	
8. Constitution	Carbonitrogenoid (excess of carbon and nitrogen).	Hydrogenoid (excess of water).	Oxygenoid (excess of oxygen).	Changeable constitution with alternation and periodicity.
9. Psychic Manifestations The Person	The sterile philosopher with lots of ideas, which he cannot materialise. Psora is theoretical but has no sense of practicality. Dishonesty, secretiveness, wickedness and impurity play a good part in him.	Sycosis is deceitful, sullen and cunning and has a tendency to exploit others. A very practical person that always cares for their own benefit and pleasures above others.	An urge for destruction seems to be the only emotion of the syphilitic person. They lack a sense of realisation, duty and understanding. Committed criminals and cold-blooded murderers are syphilitic. Their mentality vitiates the sense of judgement.	Dissatisfaction, changeability, and a lack of tolerance and perseverance are tubercular.

Key Word	Psora Sensitising Miasm	Sycosis Miasm of Incoordination	Syphilis Degenerating Miasm	Tubercular Responsive, Reactive Miasm
Nature of the Miasm	Psora is the sensitising miasm for its hyperactive and hypersensitive mind and body, which results from hypo-immunity and increased susceptibility.	Sycosis is 'hyper', and the miasm of incoordinations. This manifests as hyper abnormal behaviours or mental incoordinations such as extreme jealousy, loquacity and selfishness.	Syphilis is the miasm of destruction, destroying the love of one's own life and resulting in self-destruction or the killing of others. Syphilitics therefore have suicidal tendencies or can be cold-blooded murderers. They may be called iconoclasts and have a total lack of mercy and sympathy.	The tubercular miasm is one of changeableness. A dissatisfied state of mind makes the subject changeable both mentally and physically.
Work	Quickly fatigued with desire to lie down is characteristic of psora. The patient is indolent.	The sycotic patient is a hyper-workaholic.	The syphilitic patient is disinterested in work due to their lack of realisation and understanding.	Changeableness and impatience make it hard for the tubercular patient to concentrate on work.
Behaviour	Psora is fearful, anxious, alert and apprehensive.	Sycosis is quarrelsome, jealous, selfish and cunning with a tendency to harm (emotionally) others and animals. Ostentation and fatuousness are sycotic tendencies. The subject is often suspicious of his own works and his surroundings. Mischievous, mean and selfish summarise the sycotic psychic essence.	Syphilis is cruel and destructive and often does bodily harm to himself and others.	Fearlessness and an absolute lack of anxiety are denominating features of the tubercular miasm. There is a careless, unconcerned or indifferent attitude towards the seriousness of their sufferings and they are always hopeful of a recovery.

Key Word	Psora Sensitising Miasm	Sycosis Miasm of Incoordination	Syphilis Degenerating Miasm	Tubercular Responsive, Reactive Miasm
Memory	Weakness of memory indicates psora.	Absentmindedness is sycotic. The patient loses the thread of the conversation and forgets the recent events although they can remember past events well.	Forgetfulness is syphilitic. There is a mental paralysis where the patient reads but cannot retain the information. The mind is slow.	Changeableness of thought and perception is tubercular.
Death	It is only the psoric miasm which fears death. There is often much anxiety and an anticipation towards death.	Men and women who commit suicide today are mainly syphilo-sycotic. Sycotics will plan their own death but too many attachments and an urge to live make it difficult for them to really commit suicide.	The syphilitic patient dwells on suicide, has suicidal dreams and thoughts and an actual urge to commit suicide. Love for their own life is destroyed.	Dissatisfaction with their own life, changeableness and a vagabond mentality lead to suicidal impulses in the tubercular patient. An instinct towards self-destruction is characterised by carelessness.
Selfishness & Deprivation	Psora, by dint of its selfish nature has a tendency to deprive others (a characteristic which is also strongly present in sycosis). Deprivation exists in the sense of presenting a false or pseudo image of himself. Psoric patients may donate (although not voluntarily) a large sum of money to charity but they will ensure that they receive some personal benefit from their action.	In all varieties of deprivation and rudeness sycosis is present. The sycotic patient's prime concern is for his or her own benefit, and they will act selfishly to deprive others in order to achieve this end.	Syphilitic patients rarely deprive others as their lack of realisation extends to that of their own benefit. They are selfish only in the sense of being focussed in one particular direction, e.g. with destructive impulse, they forget or ignore everything else around them.	Extreme irritability and outrageousness with a lack of tolerance can be reflected as the selfish nature of the tubercular miasm.

Key Word	Psora Sensitising Miasm	Sycosis Miasm of Incoordination	Syphilis Degenerating Miasm	Tubercular Responsive, Reactive Miasm
Fear	All varieties of fears are classified as psoric and in this miasm they manifest as anxiety, alertness and apprehension of impending misfortune. Mental restlessness is one of the expressions of psoric fear.	As a result of incoordination of thoughts, sycosis does manifest some fears. A millionaire, for example, may develop a constant fear of poverty, which is expressed as selfishness, suspiciousness and physical restlessness.	The syphilitic lack of realisation and expression means that their fears are not properly manifested. They are close-mouthed and the only possible outward feature one might expect from a syphilitic person is of anguish.	Fearlessness is characteristic of tubercular miasm and this is well expressed by the patient as a complete indifference towards their health. Their only real fear is of dogs or other animals.
Expression	Psora is full of ideas and philosophical expression. There may be piles of books on the table and the person will go from book to book, reading only superficially. There is no depth, various ideas crowd the mind and there is no practicality at all. This constant flow of ideas is as a result of the mental restlessness.	Jealousy and suspicion are very evident in sycotic expression, and there is a tendency to suppress and conceal. This deep suspicion means that the patient does not trust anything and checks everything many times.	The syphilitic patient is an introvert, a close-mouthed fellow who keeps his depression inside and the first thing anyone knows of it is when he has committed suicide. There is also a suppressive tendency to conceal and an inability to realise and express symptoms. These patients want to escape from themselves, as well as from others, and idiocy, ignorance and obstinacy lead to melancholia and gloominess.	In the tubercular miasm, mental symptoms, especially anger are aggravated after sleep and the patient may wake with a look of dissatisfaction clearly manifested on their face. Changeability, lack of tolerance and impatience sum up the expressions of the tubercular miasm.
10. Key Words of Mental Manifestations	i) Anxious and fearful. ii) Philosophical.	i) Suspicious and jealous. ii) Arrogant.	i) Destructive and melancholic. ii) Close-mouthed.	i) Changeable and fearless. ii) Indifferent.

Key Word	Psora Sensitising Miasm	Sycosis Miasm of Incoordination	Syphilis Degenerating Miasm	Tubercular Responsive, Reactive Miasm
	iii) Irritability with anxiety.	iii) Irritability explodes into anger. The subject may bang the table, throw things and become generally restless.	iii) Irritability with cruelty.	iii) Irritability with impatience.
	iv) Sadness.	iv) Moaning.	iv) Lamenting.	iv) Changeable mood.
	v) Nervous.	v) Chaos = Syco-syphilo-psora.	v) Madness = Syphilo-syco-psora.	v) Insanity (recurrent and periodical) = Mixed miasmatic with tubercular preponderance.
	vi) Thoughtful but no practical sense.	vi) Thoughtfulness focussed for their own personal benefit.	vi) Vanishing of thoughts.	vi) Changeability of thoughts.
	vii) Lack of concentration. Weakness of memory.	vii) Incoordination in concentration, absentmindedness.	vii) Total destruction of concentration; forgetful. Dullness = weak perception.	vii) Changeability of concentration.
	viii) Malicious = Psora-syphilo-sycotic.	viii) Mischievous = Syco-syphilo-psora.	viii) Hatred = Syphilo-syco-psora.	viii) Indifferent.
	ix) Wariness of life = Psora-syphilitic.	ix) Tendency to exploit everything from life = sycotic.	ix) Loathing of life = Syphilo-psoric.	ix) Unfulfilling life.
	x) Illusions.	x) Delusions.	x) Hallucinations and deliriums.	x) Vacillation of thoughts.
	xi) Sad and depressed.	xi) Irascible, rude, ill-mannered.	xi) Sentimental and close-mouthed.	xi) Independent and indifferent.

Key Word	Psora Sensitising Miasm	Sycosis Miasm of Incoordination	Syphilis Degenerating Miasm	Tubercular Responsive, Reactive Miasm
	xii) Psora plans a robbery, has plenty of ideas but there are lots of loopholes in the plan.	xii) Sycosis is cunning and practical, fills up the loopholes and appears to hide from the actual site of the crime. He is there however and ends up with the spoils, depriving the others of their share.	xii) Syphilis is the hired criminal at the forefront of the crime. He has the inability to realise that if he is caught he will go to prison and there will be no one to look after his family!	xii) The tubercular criminal is changeable and undependable and although he commits to joining this bank robbery, he changes his mind at the last moment and does not turn up.
	xiii) Psoric memory is poor but the patient is very studious. Once they have learnt a subject they will remember it.	xiii) Sycotics have an active memory and record everything — the journalist type.	xiii) Syphilitics do not remember recent happenings but retain remote incidents in chronological order.	xiii) Tuberculars are careless. They are intelligent and bright but make careless mistakes.
11. Hair	i) Hair falls out after acute fevers.	i) Alopecia in circular spots.	i) Dandruff with thick yellow crusts (can be tubercular also).	i) Breaks, splits and sticks together.
	ii) Dry, lustreless, difficult to comb.	ii) Immature greyish hair.	ii) Falls in bunches. Falling hair from eyebrows, eyelashes and beard.	ii) A thick yellow heavy crust is apt to be tubercular (or syphilitic).
	iii) Splits at ends.	iii) Fishy odour from hair.	iii) Moist, gluey and greasy with an offensive odour.	
	iv) Bran-like dandruff.		iv) Ingrowing hair of eyelashes.	
12. Vertigo	Vertigo from indigestion or emotional disturbances.	Vertigo from closing the eyes, disappearing on opening the eyes.	Vertigo occurring at night.	Vertigo begins at the base of the brain.

Key Word	Psora Sensitising Miasm		Sycosis Miasm of Incoordination		Syphilis Degenerating Miasm		Tubercular Responsive, Reactive Miasm	
13. Eye	i)	Visualises various colours (spots before the eyes).	i)	Aggravated from changes of season and rainy weather.	i)	Structural eye changes.	i)	Red lids (Psora-tubercular).
			ii)	Ptosis.	ii)	Deformities of lens; all varieties of refractory changes. Weakness, ptosis (syphilis & sycosis).	ii)	Photophobia.
							iii)	Aversion to artificial lights.
14. Ear	i)	Dry and scaly meatus even in otorrhoea. On looking at the meatus one finds dryness immediately following the discharge.	i)	Thickening of the ear (pinna).	i)	Long ears.	i)	Acute suppurative otitis media developing as a result of some severe disease such as measles or scarlet fever offers a good prognosis in the tubercular miasm.
	ii)	Oversensitive to noise.	ii)	Growths and anatomical incoordination over the external ear.			ii)	Colds and sore throats result in acute suppurative otitis media with offensive pus.
15. Nose	i)	Sensitive to odours.	i)	Nasal congestion ameliorated even by the slightest amount of nasal discharges (abnormal discharge ameliorates).	i)	Ulceration of nasal septum.	i)	Epistaxis.

Key Word	Psora Sensitising Miasm	Sycosis Miasm of Incoordination	Syphilis Degenerating Miasm	Tubercular Responsive, Reactive Miasm
	ii) Psoric cold begins with sneezing, redness and heat. The nose becomes sensitive to touch when it is continually blown.	ii) A bland or acidic discharge from the nose with a fish-brine smell is characteristic.	ii) Diminution of sense of smell.	ii) Recurrent catching of colds.
	iii) Redness of mucous membranes.			iii) Flushing of nose.
16. Mouth	i) Tartar.	i) Fishy taste.	i) Ulcers in the oral cavity.	i) Taste of pus.
	ii) All food tastes as if burnt is a characteristic.		ii) Asymmetrical teeth.	ii) Bright red, bleeding from gums.
	iii) Refuses highly aromatic substances.		iii) Tongue having the imprint of the teeth.	
	iv) Intolerable sweet taste in mouth.		iv) Saliva is offensive, and can be drawn into threads.	
			v) Coppery or metallic taste.	
			vi) Crowns of incisors are crescentic.	
17. Face	i) Inverted.	i) Dropsical.	i) Oily, greasy face.	i) Sunken eyes and pale face but flushed cheeks.
	ii) Blue — cyanosis due to lack of oxygenation. Blue, the cold colour represents psora.	ii) Yellowish complexion. The colour yellow corresponds to sycosis.	ii) High cheek bones and rough skin.	ii) Round faced with fair, smooth, clear skin and a waxy smoothness of complexion.

Key Word	Psora Sensitising Miasm		Sycosis Miasm of Incoordination		Syphilis Degenerating Miasm		Tubercular Responsive, Reactive Miasm	
					iii)	Face looks puckered, dried and wrinkled like that of an old person.	iii)	The face looks well even in the last stages of disease when the rest of the body has become emaciated.
					iv)	Thick lips.	iv)	Thin lips.
					v)	Eyelids red and inflamed.	v)	Eyes are bright and sparkling.
					vi)	Scaly, crusty lashes; broken, shabby, irregularly curved and imperfect.	vi)	Eyebrows and lashes are soft, glossy, long and silken.
18. Heart & Pulse	i)	Psoric heart patients worry about their conditions; take their pulse frequently; fear death; remain quiet.	i)	A combination of sycosis and psora provides the right soil for valvular and cardiac disturbances.	i)	High blood pressure where the systolic and diastolic pressures are irregularly distributed, e.g. high systolic combined with a low diastolic rate.	i)	Palpitations, which are aggravated by higher altitudes. The patient wants to keep still and is unable to climb stairs or ascend hills.
	ii)	Bradycardia.	ii)	Tachycardia.	ii)	Irregular pulse.	ii)	The pulse is feeble but rapid.
	iii)	Hammering sensation in pericardium.	iii)	Rheumatic and valvular heart diseases.				
	iv)	Hypotension.	iv)	Hypertension.				
			v)	Hypertrophy of the heart.				

Key Word	Psora Sensitising Miasm	Sycosis Miasm of Incoordination	Syphilis Degenerating Miasm	Tubercular Responsive, Reactive Miasm
19. Abdomen	i) Slow intestinal peristalsis.	i) Accelerated and exaggerated peristalsis. ii) Children born of sycotic parents suffer from colic, almost from the moment of birth. Sycotic children are subject to colic and "three-month's colic".	i) Irregular peristalsis resulting in spasm associated with dysentery.	i) Duodenal ulcers.
20. Stool	i) Constipation is primarily psoric. ii) Offensive stool, not very painful. iii) Stool may be of any colour. iv) Worse from cold, motion, and eating and drinking cold things. Better by warm drinks, hot food, and warm applications to the abdomen.	i) Diarrhoea is sycotic. ii) Diarrhoea gushes and ejaculates forcefully and is colicky in nature. iii) Sour, acrid, grass green stool. iv) Jet like expulsion of faeces, with a sense of insecurity and a constant symptom of griping.	i) Dysentery is syphilitic. ii) Stool is mixed with lots of mucus, scrapings of intestine, and sometimes blood.	i) Morning diarrhoea with extreme prostration and debility is tubercular. ii) Bleeding from the rectum with or without stool.

Key Word	Psora Sensitising Miasm	Sycosis Miasm of Incoordination	Syphilis Degenerating Miasm	Tubercular Responsive, Reactive Miasm
21. Skin	i) Persistent dryness.	i) Painful with pains better by pressure.	i) Ulcerous tendency — open ulcers of virulent type.	i) Skin diseases, which are threatening or destructive in nature.
	ii) Suppression of skin conditions directly affects the mind.	ii) Suppression of skin diseases affects firstly the nerve centres, followed by the heart, liver and reproductive system.	ii) When syphilitic skin is suppressed the intellect is affected causing dullness, depression and a lack of enthusiasm.	ii) Suppression of skin conditions affects the inner tissues causing destructive and ulcerous tendencies; and the deeper tissues causing a debilitated tubercular state.
	iii) Unhealthy skin with itching and burning represents psora.	iii) Oily skin with redness at the tip of the nose and copious perspiration is sycotic.	iii) Ulcerated skin with pus and blood represents syphilis.	iii) Recurrent and obstinate boils with profuse pus are tubercular.
	iv) Eruptions characterised by roughness and unwashability of the skin.	iv) Sycosis has vesicular eruptions.	iv) Copper coloured eruptions are syphilitic. Eruptions are slow to heal (psora-syphilitic).	iv) History of ringworm and the state caused by the suppression of ringworm.
	v) Skin diseases, which spread over the body.	v) Skin conditions appear localised and/or in circumscribed spots.	v) Putridity, acridity and offensiveness of all discharges.	v) Busy and important areas are affected.
		vi) Post operative scar tumours and abscesses.	vi) Stitch abscesses.	

Key Word	Psora Sensitising Miasm		Sycosis Miasm of Incoordination		Syphilis Degenerating Miasm		Tubercular Responsive, Reactive Miasm	
			vii)	Disturbed pigment metabolism produces hyper-pigmentation and depigmentation in patches or diffused in different parts. Patches may be urine coloured.				
22. Nails	i)	Dry, harsh appearance of the nails.	i)	Irregular nails, ridged or ribbed, or ridged and corrugated.	i)	Spoon-shaped.	i)	Fissured, wavy, asymmetrical nails, which come out easily.
			ii)	Thick.	ii)	Paper-like, thin nails which bend and tear easily.	ii)	Irregular nails, break and split easily.
			iii)	Pale.	iii)	Whitlows are psora-syphilitic (like other periosteal inflammations).	iii)	Nails with various stains and spots or with white specks and scalloped edges.
			iv)	Convex appearance.	iv)	Concave appearance.	iv)	Glossy nails.
							v)	Formation of pus at the junction of nails and flesh with severe stitching pains.
							vi)	The natural convexity is often reversed.
							vii)	Hangnails.

Key Word	Psora Sensitising Miasm	Sycosis Miasm of Incoordination	Syphilis Degenerating Miasm	Tubercular Responsive, Reactive Miasm
23. Pains	i) Psoric neuralgic pains are usually better by quiet, rest and warmth, and worse by motion.	i) The rheumatic pains of sycosis are worse by cold and damp, and better by moving or stretching.	i) Bone pains are syphilitic.	i) Sense of great exhaustion, patient tires easily and never seems to get rested. As the sun ascends their strength revives a little, as it descends, they lose it again.
	ii) Sore, bruised, pressive pains are psoric.	ii) Joint pains are sycotic and pains are generally stitching, pulsating or wandering.	ii) Burning, bursting and tearing pains are syphilitic.	
24. Malignancy	i) Prone to develop at the age of 40.	i) Prone to develop at any age.	i) Prone to develop at the age of 40.	i) Tubercular malignancies are characterised by metastasis and haemorrhage.
	ii) Prefers tissues of ectodermal origin.	ii) Prefers tissues of entodermal origin.	ii) Prefers tissues of mesodermal origin.	
	iii) Hahnemann says in Chronic Diseases that even large sarcomatous lesions can develop from psora.	iii) Sycotic malignant tumours are encapsulated and grow out of proportion. There is incoordination in cellular proliferation.	iii) Syphilitic malignant tumours break open their capsules causing degeneration, disintegration and cellular necrosis.	

Key Word	Psora Sensitising Miasm	Sycosis Miasm of Incoordination	Syphilis Degenerating Miasm	Tubercular Responsive, Reactive Miasm
25. Desires & Aversions	Desires: Sweet, sour, fatty, fried, indigestible, spicy, oily and hot foods.	Desires: Table salt, alcohol, coconut, fatty meat, peppers, pungent, well-seasoned foods and salty foods. The patient craves beer (which causes less aggravation than wine).	Desires: Stimulants — alcohol, tea, coffee, smoking (all signs of destruction), very spicy meat, cold food and sour things. Desires foods, which are either too hot or too cold.	Desires: Indigestible things like clay etc., and fatty, greasy foods on which they thrive. Crave the things, which make them sick. Desires potatoes, tea, tobacco and meat and crave salt which they will eat alone from the saucer. Tuberculars are extremists and like either very hot or really cold things.
	Aversions: Milk, boiled food and cold foods.	Aversions: Meat and wine, which aggravate the sycotic condition, milk, and spices of which they are intolerant.	Aversions: Meat, especially less spicy, and other animal foods.	Aversions: meat (generally desire for meat is strongest but due to the changeability of the miasm, aversion may also occur). The tubercular patient does not digest starches easily.
26. Modalities	Aggravated by standing and from cold. Wants warmth externally and internally and is therefore worse in winter.	Aggravated by rest, damp, rainy, humid atmospheres, during thunderstorms, changes of weather, and from meat.	Aggravated from sunset to sunrise, movement, extremes of temperature, at the seaside, on sea-voyages, and from thunderstorms.	Aggravated from thunderstorm, night, milk, fruits, greasy and oily foods.
	Aggravated between sunrise and sunset.	The sycotic patient is a barometer — when it rains, he has pains and he suffers.	Aggravated by warmth, during the summer, at night, from the warmth of the bed and from sweat (through natural discharges).	Aggravated in closed room. Patient also cannot tolerate any pressure in the chest.

Key Word	Psora Sensitising Miasm	Sycosis Miasm of Incoordination	Syphilis Degenerating Miasm	Tubercular Responsive, Reactive Miasm
	Ameliorated in summer, from heat, by natural discharges such as urine, menstruation etc. Ameliorated through physiological eliminative processes such as sweat.	Ameliorated from motion, unnatural discharges (which are generally greenish/yellow in colour) and unnatural eliminations through the mucus surfaces, e.g. leucorrhoea, nasal discharge etc. Physiological eliminations do not ameliorate.	Amelioration from sunrise to sunset, change of position, a lukewarm climate, and from any abnormal discharges (such as leucorrhoea, coryza).	Ameliorated in dry weather, open air, and during the daytime.
	Ameliorated by hot application, scratching, crying and eating.	Amelioration by slow motion, or by stretching, in dry weather, lying on stomach or by pressure. The return of suppressed normal discharges such as menses also ameliorate.	Amelioration during winter, from cold in winter.	Temporarily ameliorated by offensive foot or axillary sweat which when suppressed induces lung trouble.
	The appearance of suppressed skin eruptions ameliorates.	Ameliorated when warts or fibrous growths appear.	Amelioration through the discharge of pus (if old ulcers open up).	Ameliorated by nose bleeding.
		Ameliorated in general from the return or breaking open of old ulcers or sores, and markedly ameliorated by the return of acute gonorrhoeal manifestations.		Tubercular modalities depend upon the preponderance of the psoric or syphilitic miasm.

PART — II

MIASMATIC DIAGNOSIS :
MIASMATIC WEIGHTAGE OF MEDICINES

Medicine	Psoric	Sycotic	Syphilitic	Tubercular	Chilly or Hot
ABIES CANADENSIS	++	+	+	++	C++
ABIES NIGRA	++	+	+	+	
ABROTANUM	++	+++		++	C+
ABSINTHIUM	++	+	++	+	
ACALYPHA INDICA	++	+		+++	C++
ACETANILIDUM	++	++	+	+	C++
ACETIC ACID	++	+	+	+++	C+
ACONITUM NAPELLUS	++	+	+	++	C+
ACTAEA RACEMOSA	+	+++	+	+	C+
ACTEA SPICATA	++	+++	++	+	
ADONIS VERNALIS	++	++	+	++	
ADRENALIN	++	++	+	+	
AESCULUS HIPPOCASTANUM	++	++	+	+	H++
AETHUSA CYNAPIUM	++	+	+	+	H+
AGARICUS MUSCARIUS	+	++	+	+++	C+++
AGNUS CASTUS	+	+++	+	+	C+
AILANTHUS GLANDULOSA	+	++	+	+++	
ALETRIS FARINOSA	++	+	+	+	C++
ALFALFA	++	++		++	
ALLIUM CEPA	++	++	+	++	H++
ALLIUM SATIVUM	++	+	+	+++	C+
ALNUS	++	++	+	++	
ALOE SOCOTRINA	++	++	+	++	H++
ALSTONIA SCHOLARIS	++	+	+	+	
ALUMINA	++	++	+	+	C+++
ALUMINA SILICATA	++	+	++	+	C++
AMBRA GRISEA	+	+	+	++	C+
AMBROSIA	++	+	+	++	
AMMONIUM BENZOICUM	++	+++			
AMMONIUM BROMATUM	++	++			
AMMONIUM CARBONICUM	++	+		+++	C+
AMMONIUM CAUSTICUM	++		++	+++	C++
AMMONIUM IODATUM	++	++			
AMMONIUM MURIATICUM	++	++		+	H+
AMMONIUM PHOSPHORICUM	++	+++			
AMYLENUM NITROSUM	++		+	+	H++
ANACARDIUM	++	++	++	+	H+
ANAGALLIS	++	+++	+	+	
ANATHERUM	++	++	++	+	
ANGUSTURA VERA	++	+++	+++	++	C+
ANTHRACINUM	++	+	+++	+	
ANTHRAKOKALI	++	++	+	++	
ANTIMONIUM ARSENICOSUM	++	++	+	+	C+
ANTIMONIUM CRUDUM	++	++	+	+	C+
ANTIMONIUM TARTARICUM	++	++	+	+	H++
APIS MELLIFICA	+	+++	+	+	C+
APOCYNUM CANNABINUM	++	+	++	+	
APOMORPHIA	++	+	++		
ARAGALLUS LAMBERTI	+	++	+	+	
ARALIA RACEMOSA	++	++	+	++	
ARANEA DIADEMA	++	+++	+	++	C+++
ARBUTUS ANDRACHNE	++	+++			
ARGEMONE MEXICANA	++	++			
ARGENTICUM METALLICUM	+	++	++	+	H+
ARGENTICUM NITRICUM	+++	+++	+++	+++	H++

118

L denotes leading remedies within each miasm.

L denotes leading remedies within each miasm.

Medicine	Psoric	Sycotic	Syphilitic	Tubercular	Chilly or Hot
ARNICA MONTANA	++	++	++	+++	C+
ARSENICUM ALBUM	+++	+++	+	++	C+++
ARSENICUM BROMATUM	++	+	+++	+	H++
ARSENICUM IODATUM	+++				C++
ARSENICUM METALLICUM	++	+		+++ L	
ARSENICUM SULF. FLAVUM	++	+		++	H+
ARTEMISIA VULGARIS	++				
ARUM TRIPHYLLUM	++				C+
ARUNDO	++	+	+++	++	
ASAFOETIDA	++	+	+++	+	C++
ASARUM EUROPUM	++		++		H++
ASCLEPIAS TUBEROSA	++	++	+	+	C++
ASIMINA TRILOBA	++	+	++		
ASPARAGUS OFFICINALIS	+	++	++	++	
ASPIDOSPERMA	++	++			
ASTACUS FLUVIATILIS	++	+	+	+	C+
ASTERIAS RUBENS	+	+++	+++		C+
AURUM METALLICUM	++	++	+++ L	++	C++
AURUM MUR. NATRONATUM	+++	+++	++	+	
AVENA SATIVA	+++	+	+		
AZADIRACHTA INDICA	++	++	+		C+
BACILLINUM	++	+++	++	+++ L	H+
BADIAGA	++	++	+	++	C++
BALSAMUM PERUVIANUM	++	+++	+	++	H++
BAPTISIA TINCTORIA	++	++		+++	H+
BARYTA CARBONICUM	+++	++	++	+++	C++
BELLADONNA	+		+	+++	H++
BENZOICUM ACIDUM	+++	+++		+++	C+
BERBERIS VULGARIS	+	+++		+	C+
BORAX	++	++	+	++	H++
BOVISTA	++	+		++	H++
BROMIUM	+	+		++	H++
BRYONIA ALBA	++	+++	+	+++	H+
CACTUS GRANDIFLORUS	++	++		++	C++
CALADIUM	+	+		+	C++
CALCAREA ARSENICA	++	+++	++	+++ L	C++
CALCAREA CARBONICA	+++ L	+++	++	+++	C++
CALCAREA IODATA	++	+++	+	+++	H++
CALCAREA PHOSPHORICA	+	+	++	+++	C++
CALCAREA SULPHURICA	++	+	+++	++	H++
CALENDULA	++	++	+++	+	C+
CAMPHORA	++	+	+	++	C++
CANNABIS INDICA	++	++			H++
CANNABIS SATIVA	++	+++	+++	++	C+
CANTHARIDES	++	+++	+++	++	C+
CAPSICUM	+++	+	+	++	C+++
CARBO ANIMALIS	+	++	+++	+++	C++
CARBO VEGETABILIS	+++	+	++	+++	C++
CARBOLIC ACID	++	+	++	+	C+
CAULOPHYLLUM	+++	+++	++	++	C+
CAUSTICUM	+++	+++	++	+++	C++
CHAMOMILLA	++	++	++	+	H++
CHELIDONIUM MAJUS	+++	+	+++	+	C+
CICUTA VIROSA	++		++	+	C+
CINA	++		+	++	H+
CINCHONA OFFICINALIS	++	++	+	+++	C++
CINNABARIS	++	+	++	++	C+
CISTUS CANADENSIS	++	+	+++	+++	C++
CLEMATIS	+	+	+	+	C++
COCA	++	+	++	++	C+
COCCULUS	++	+	++	++	C++
COCCUS CACTI	+			.	C++
COFFEA	++	++		+	C++

Medicine	Psoric	Sycotic	Syphilitic	Tubercular	Chilly or Hot
COLCHICUM	++	++	+		C+
COLLINSONIA CANADENSIS	++	++		++	C+
COLOCYNTHIS	++	++	+		C+
CONIUM MACULATUM	++	++	+	+	C++
CROCUS SATIVA	++			++	H+
CROTALUS HORRIDUS	++	++	+	+++	H+
CROTON TIGLIUM	++	+	+	+	H+
CUPRUM METALLICUM	++	++	++	+	C++
CYCLAMEN EUROPAEUM	++	++		++	C++
DIGITALIS PURPUREA	++	++		+	C++
DIOSCOREA VILLOSA	++	++			H+
DIPHTHERINUM	++	+	+	++	C++
DROSERA ROTUNDIFOLIA	++	+	+	++	C++
DULCAMARA	++	++	+	+	C++
EQUISETUM HYEMALE	++	++			C+
EUPATORIUM PERFOLIATUM	++	+	+	++	C+
EUPHRASIA	++	+	+	+	H+
FERRUM METALLICUM	++	++	+	++	C+
FERRUM PHOSPHORICUM	++	+	+	++	C++
FLUORICUM ACIDUM	++	+	+++	++	H++
GELSEMIUM	+	++	+	+	H++
GLONOINE	++	+	+	++	H++
GRAPHITES	+++	++		++	C+++
GUN POWDER	++	++	+++ L	++	C++
HAMAMELIS VIRGINICA	++	+	+	+++	H+
HELLEBORUS	++	+++	+	++	C+
HEPAR SULPHURIS	+++	++	++	+++	C+++
HYDRASTIS	++	++	+++	++	C+
HYDROPHOBINUM (LYSSINUM)	++	++	+++	++	C++
HYOSCYAMUS	++	+++	+	++	C+
HYPERICUM	+++	++	++	++	C+
IBERIS	++	+	+	+++	C+
IGNATIA	+++	++	+	+++	C+
IODUM	++	+	++	+++ L	H+++
IPECACUANHA	++	+	++	+++	C+
IRIS VERSICOLOR	++	+	++	++	H+
JATROPHA	++	+	+	++	
JUGULANS CINEREA	++	++		++	C+
JUSTICIA ADHATODA	++	+		++	C++
KALI ARSENICUM	++	++	+++	+	C++
KALI BICHROMICUM	++	++	+++	++	C++
KALI BROMATUM	++	++	+	++	
KALI CARBONICUM	++	++	+	+++	C+++
KALI IOD (HYDRIODICUM)	++	++	+++	+	H+
KALI MURIATICUM	++	+	+	++	C+
KALI PHOSPHORICUM	++	++	++	+	C+
KALI SILICATUM	++	++	+	++	C++
KALI SULPHURICUM	++	+++	+	++	H++
KALMIA LATIFOLIA	++	+++	+	++	C+
KOUSSO	++	+	+++ L	++	
KREOSOTUM	+++	+	+++ L	++	C++
LAC CANINUM	++	+	+	++	H+
LAC DEFLORATUM	++	+		+	C+
LACHESIS	++	+++	++	+++	H++
LACHNANTHES	++	++		++	
LACTICUM ACIDUM	++	+	+	++	C+
LACTUCA VIROSA	+	++			H+
LAMIUM	+	++	+	+	
LAPIS ALBUS	++	+++	+	++	
LAPPA	++	++	+	+	
LATHYRUS	++	+	+		C+
LATRODECTUS MACTANS	++	+			
LAUROCERASUS	++	+		+	H+

120

L denotes leading remedies within each miasm.

Medicine	Psoric	Sycotic	Syphilitic	Tubercular	Chilly or Hot
LECITHIN	++				
LEDUM PAL	++			++	H++
LEMNA MINOR	++			+	C+
LEPTANDRA	+			+	C+
LILIUM TIGRINUM	++	++	+	+++	H+
LILIUM	++		+		
LIMULUS	++	++			
LITHIUM CARBONICUM	++	+++	+	+	H+
LOBELIA INFLATA	+++	++			C+
LOLIUM TEMULENTUM	++	++	+		
LUPULUS	++	++			
LUPULUS	++	+++	++	+++	C++
LYCOPODIUM	+++ L	+++	+	++	C+
LYCOPUS VIRGINICUS	+++	++	+	++	C+
MAGNESIS CARBONICA	+++	++	+	++	H+
MAGNESIA MURIATICA	++	++	+	++	C++
MAGNESIA PHOSPHORICA	++	+++	+	++	H+
MAGNESIA SULPHURICA	++	++	+	+	H+
MAGNOLIA GRANDIFLORA	++	++	+	+	C+
MALANDRINUM	++	++	++	+	H+
MANCINELLA	++	+++	++	++	C++
MANGANUM ACETICUM	++	++	+++	+++	C++
MANGIFERA INDICA	++	+	++	+++	
MEDORRHINUM	+++	+++ L	++	++	H++
MELILOTUS	++	++	+	++	H+
MENISPERNUM	++	+++	+	+	
MENYANTHES	++	++	+	+	
MEPHITIS	+++	+++	+	+	
MERCURIUS SOLUBILIS	+++	++	+++ L	+++	C++
MERCURIUS CORROSIVUS	+++	+++	+++	++	C++
MERCURIUS CYANATUS	++	++	+++	+++	C++
MERCURIUS DULCIS	++	+++	++	+++	C++
MERCURIUS IODATUS FLAVUS	++	+++	+++	+++	C++
MERCURIUS IODATUS RUBER	++	+++	+++	++	C++
MERCURIUS SULPHURICUS	++	+++	+++	++	C+++
MEZEREUM	++	++	+++ L	++	
MILLEFOLIUM	++	++	++	++	
MOMORDICA BALSAMINA	++	++	+++	++	C+
MORPHINUM	++	++	+++	+++	
MOSCHUS	++	+++	++	++	C+
MUREX	++	+++	+++	+++	C+
MURIATIC ACID	++	+++	+++	+++	C+
MYGALE LASIODARA	++	+++	+	+	
MYRICA	++	+++	+++	+	
MYRISTICA SEIBIFERA	++	+	+++	+++	H++
NAJA TRIPUDIANS	++	++	++	+++	
NARCISSUS	++	++	+	+	
NATRUM ARSENICUM	++	++	+	+	C+
NATRUM CARBONICUM	++	++	+		H+
NATRUM MURIATICUM	+++	+++	++	++	H++
NATRUM NITRICUM	++	+++	+	+++	
NATRUM PHOSPHORICUM	++	++		++	H+
NATRUM SALICYLICUM	++	++		+++	
NATRUM SULPHURICUM	++	+++ L		+	C+
NICCOLUM	++	++		++	
NITRIC ACID	++	+++ L	+++ L	+++	C+
NITRI SPIRITUS DULCIS	++	+++		+	C++
NUPHAR LUTEUM	+++	++	+	+	
NUX MOSCHATA	+++	++	+	++	C++
NUX VOMICA	+++	++	+	++	C+++
NYCTANTHES ARBOR-TRISTIS	+++	++		++	C+++
OCIMUM CANUM	++	++	+		
OENANTHE CROCATA	++	++	++	+	C++
OLEANDER	++	++			
OLEUM ANIMALE	++	+	+	+	H+

L denotes leading remedies within each miasm.

Medicine	Psoric	Sycotic	Syphilitic	Tubercular	Chilly or Hot
OLEUM JECORIS ASELLI	++	+	++	+++	C++
OLEUM SANTALI	++	+++		+	
ONOSMODIUM	++	++	+	++	
OOPHORINUM	++	+++		++	
OPERCULINA TURPETHUM	++	+++	++	++	
OPIUM	+++	++	++	+	H++
OREODAPHNE	++	++			
ORIGANUM	++	+++		+	
ORNITHOGALUM UMBELLATUM	++	++	+++	+	C+
OSMIUM	++	++	+	++	
OSTRYA VIRGINICA	++	+++			
OVI GALLINAE PELLICULA	++	++		+	
OXALICUM ACIDUM	++	++	+	+++	C+
OXYDENDRON	++	+++			
OXYTROPIS	++	+	+		
PAEONIA	++	++	+++	++	C++
PALLADIUM	++	+++	++	++	
PARAFFINE	+++	++	++	++	
PAREIRA BRAVA	++	+++	+	+	
PARIS QUADRIFOLIA	++	++	+	++	
PASSIFLORA INCARNATA	++	+++	++	+++	
PAULLINIA SORBILIS	++	+	+	++	
PENTHORUM	++	+++	+	+	
PERTUSSIN	++	++	+	+	
PETROLEUM	+++	++	++	++	C++
PETROSELINUM	++	+++	++		
PHASEOLUS	++	++		++	
PHELLANDRIUM	++	++		+++	C++
PHOSPHORICUM ACIDUM	++	++	+	+++L	C+
PHOSPHORUS	+++	+++	+++	+++L	C+++
PHYSALIS	++	+++	+	++	C++
PHYSOSTIGMA	++	++	+++	++	H+
PHYTOLACCA	++	++	+++L	++	C++
PICRIC ACID	++	++	+	+	H++
PILOCARPUS	++	++	+	+++	H+
PINUS SYLVESTRIS	++	++	+	++	
PIPER METHYSTICUM	++	+++	+	+	C+
PIPER NIGRUM	++	++	+	+	
PITUITRIN	++	+++		+	
PIX LIQUIDA	++	+		++	
PLANTAGO MAJOR	++	++	+	+	C+
PLATANUS OCCIDENTALIS	++	++			
PLATINA	++	+++	+	++	H+
PLUMBUM METALLICUM	++	+++	+	+	C+
PODOPHYLLUM	++	++			
POLYGONUM PUNCTATUM	++	++	++	+	C+
POPULUS CANDICANS	++	++	+	+	
POPULUS TREMULOIDES	++	++	+	++	
POTHOS FOETIDUS	++	++		+	H+
PRIMULA VERIS	++	++		+	C+
PROPYLAMIN	++	++			
PRUNUS SPINOSA	++	++		+	
PSORINUM	+++L	++	++	+++	C+++
PTELEA	++	++		+	H+
PULEX IRRITANS	++	+	+++		
PULSATILLA	++	+++L	+	++	H/C
PYROGENIUM	++	++	++	++	C+
QUERCUS GLANDIUM SPIRITUS	++	++	++		
RADIUM	++	+++L	++	+	C+
RANUNCULUS BULBOSUS	++	++	+	+	C+++
RANUNCULUS SCELERATUS	++	++	++	+	C+
RAPHANUS	++	+++		+	
RATANHIA	++	++	+++	++	

122

L denotes leading remedies within each miasm.

Medicine	Psoric	Sycotic	Syphilitic	Tubercular	Chilly or Hot
RHAMNUS CALIFORNICA	++	+++	+		
RHEUM	+++	++			C+
RHODIUM	++	+++	+		
RHODODENDRON	+++	+++		+	
RHUS AROMATICA	++	+++	++		C+
RHUS GLABRA	++	+++	+	++	
RHUS TOXICODENDRON	+++	+++	++	+	
RHUS VENENATA	++	+++	+++	++	C++
RICINUS COMMUNIS	++	++	+	++	C+
ROBINIA	+++	++			
ROSA DAMASCENA	++	++	+	++	
RUMEX CRISPUS	++	+++	+	++	C++
RUTA GRAVEOLENS	++	++	+++	+	C+
SABADILLA	+++	++	+++	+++	C+++
SABAL SERRULATA	++	+++	+	++	
SABINA	++	++	+	+++	H++
SACCHARUM OFFICINALE	++	++	++	++	
SALICYLICUM ACIDUM	++	+	+	++	C+
SALIX NIGRA	++	++	+	+	
SALVIA OFFICINALIS	+++	++	++	++	C+
SAMBUCUS NIGRA	++	++	+	++	C+
SANGUINARIA	++	+	++	+++	C+
SANGUINARIA NITRICA	+++	+++	++	+	
SANICULA	++	+++	+	+	C+
SANTONINUM	++	++		+++	
SAPONARIA	++	++	+	++	H++
SARCOLACTIC ACID	+++	++	+	++	
SARRACENIA PURPUREA	++	+			
SARSAPARILLA	++	+++	++	+	C+
SCROPHULARIA NODOSA	++	+++	++	+++	C+
SCUTELLARIA	++	++	++		
SECALE CORNUTUM	++	++	++	+++	
SEDUM ACRE	++	++	+		
SELENIUM	++	+++	+	++	H++
SEMPERVIVUM TECTORUM	++	++	++	+++	
SENECIO AUREUS	++	++	+	+	C++
SENEGA	++	++		++	C++
SENNA	++	++		++	
SEPIA	++	+++ L	+	++	C+++
SERUM ANGUILLAR (EEL SERUM)	++	+++	+++	+	
SILICEA	++	++	+++	+++ L	C+++
SINAPIS NIGRA	++	++	+	+++	
SKOOKUM CHUCK	+++	+++		+	
SOLANUM LYCOPERSICUM	++	++	++	+	C++
SOLANUM NIGRUM	++	++	+++	+++	
SOLIDAGO VIRGA	++	++		+++	
SPARTIUM SCOPARIUM	+++	++	+++	+	
SPIGELIA	+++	++	+	+++	C++
SPIRANTHES	++	+++			
SPONGIA TOSTA	++	++		++	H+
SQUILLA	++	++	++	+++	
STANNUM	+++	++	++	+++ L	C+
STAPHYSAGRIA	++	+++ L	++	++	C++
STELLARIA MEDIA	+++	++	+++ L	+	H++
STERCULIA	++	++			
STICTA	++	+++	+	++	C++
STIGMATA MAYDIS	++	+++	+++		
STILLINGIA	++	+++			C+
STRAMONIUM	++	+++	+	+	C++
STRONTIA	++	+++	+	+++	C+++
STROPHANTHUS HISPIDUS	++	++	++	+	
STRYCHNINUM	++	+++	++	+	C+
STRYCHNIA PHOSPHORICA	++	+++	+	+	

L denotes leading remedies within each miasm.

Medicine	Psoric	Sycotic	Syphilitic	Tubercular	Chilly or Hot
SUCCINUM	++	++		+	
SULFONAL	+++	+++		++	
SULPHUR	+++L	++	+++	+++	H+++
SULPHUR IODATUM	++	+++	++	+	H+++
SULPHURICUM ACIDUM	++	++	+++	+++	C++
SULPHUROSUM ACIDUM	++	++	+++	++	
SUMBUL	+++	+++	+		C+
SYMPHORICARPUS RACEMOSA	++	++		+	
SYMPHYTUM	++	++	+	+	
SYPHILINUM	+++	++	+++L	++	C++
SYZYGIUM JAMBOLANUM	+++	+	++	++	
TABACUM	++	++	+		H+
TANACETUM VULGARE	+++	++	++		
TANNIC ACID	++	+++		++	
TARENTULA CUBENSIS	++	+	+++L	++	
TARENTULA HISPANIA	++	+++	++	+++	H++
TARAXACUM	+++	+	+	+++	
TARTARICUM ACIDUM	+++	++		+++	H+
TAXUS BACCATA	++	+++	.	+++	
TELLURIUM	++	+++	++	++	C++
TEREBINTHINA	++	+++	++	+++L	C+
TEUCRIUM MARUM VARUM	+++	+++	+	++	H+
THALLIUM	++	++	++	++	
THASPIUM AUREUM	++	++	+++	.	
THEA	++	+	+	++	C++
THERIDION	++	+++	++	+++	C+
THIOSINAMINUM	++	+++	+		
THLASPI BURSA PASTORIS	++	+++		+++L	
THUJA OCCIDENTALIS	++	+++L	++	++	C+++
THYMOL	++	+++		+	
THYMUS SERPYLLUM	++	++	+	++	
THYROIDINUM	++	+++L	++	+++	C+++
TILIA EUROPA	++	++	++	+++	H++
TITANIUM	++	++	+	+++	
TONGO	++	++			
TORULA CEREVISIAE	++	+++	+	+	
TRIBULUS TERRESTRIS	++	+++		+	C+++
TRIFOLIUM PRATENSE	++	++	+++	++	H+
TRILLIUM PENDULUM	++	+++	++	+++L	
TRIOSTEUM PERFOLIATUM	++	+++	++	+	
TRINITROTOLUENE	+++	+	++	+++	
TROMBIDIUM	++	++	+++	+	
TUBERCULINUM	+++	+++	++	+++L	C+++
TURNERA	++	+++		++	
TUSSILAGO PETASITES	++	+++			
UPAS TIENTE	++	++	+	+	
URANIUM NITRICUM	++	+++	++	++	
UREA	++	++	+	+++	
URTICA URENS	++	+++L	+	+++	
USNEA BARBATA	+++	++		+	
USTILAGO MAYDIS	++	+++	+	++	
UVA URSI	++	+++	+	++	
VACCININUM	++	+++			
VALERIANA	++	.++	+	+	C+
VANADIUM	++	++	++	++	
VANILLA	++	+++		++	
VARIOLINUM	++	++	+	+++	
VERATRUM ALBUM	+++	+++	+	++	C++
VERATRUM VIRIDE	++	+++	+	++	
VERBASCUM	+++	++	+	+++	
VERBENA	++	+	++	+	
VESPA CRABRO	++	++	+	++	C++
VIBURNUM OPULUS	++	+++	+	+	H++

L denotes leading remedies within each miasm.

Medicine	Psoric	Sycotic	Syphilitic	Tubercular	Chilly or Hot
VINCA MINOR	+	+			
VIOLA ODORATA	++	+	+	++	C++
VIOLA TRICOLOR	+++	+++	+	++	C++
VISCUM ALBUM	++	+++	++	++	C+++
WYETHIA	++	++	+	++	
XANTHOXYLUM	++	++	++	+	
XEROPHYLLUM	++	++	++	++	C+
X-RAY	++	+++ L	++	++	C+
YOHIMBINUM	++	+++	+	+	
YUCCA FILAMENTOSA	++	+++	++	++	
ZINCUM METALLICUM	++	++	++	++	
ZINCUM VALERIANUM	++	+++		+	C+
ZINGIBER					

L denotes leading remedies within each miasm.

125

PART — III
MIASMATIC DIAGNOSIS:
LEADING ANTI-MIASMATIC MEDICINES

LEADING ANTI-PSORIC MEDICINES:

ALOES, *Alumina*, Ambra, Ammon.carb., Anacard, Ant.c., *Apis.mel.*, Arg.nit., *Ars. alb.*, Ars. iod., Avena sativa , Baryta.carb., *Bell*, Borax, Bryonia, Bufo.r., Calc.ars., **CALC.CARB**., Caps, Carbo veg., Causticum, Cist.c., Coc.c., Conium.mac., Cup.m., Digit, *Dulcamara*, Ferr.met., Ferr.phos., *Graph*, **HEP.SULPH**, Hypericum, *Ignatia*, Kali phos., *Kali.carb.*, Lac.c., Lach., Led., **LYCO**., *Mag.c.*, Mag.m., Mang.acet, Melilotus, Merc Cor, Merc Sol, Mur.ac. Nat.c., Natrum Mur, Nuphar Luteum, Nux Moschata, Nux Vomica, Nyctanthes, Opium, Paraffinum, Petrol, Phos, Platinum, Plumb.met., **PSORIN**, Pyrog., Rheum, Rhus tox, Robinia, Sabal ser, Sarsap., Secele cor, Selen., Silicea, Spartium Scoparium, Stan.met., Stellaria media, Sulfonal, **SULPH**., Sulph.ac. Sumbul, Syphilinum, Syzigium Jambo, Tanacetum vulgare, Taraxacum, Tarent, Tartaric acid, Teucrium marum varum., Theridon, Usnea barbata, Veratrum album, Verbascum, Vinca minor, Viola tricolor, **ZINC. MET**.

LEADING ANTI-SYCOTIC MEDICINES:

Abrotanum, Actaea racemosa, Agaricus mus., Agnus castus, Argentum met., Alumina, Ammonium benzoicum, Ammonium phosphoricum, Anacardium, Anagallis, Angustura vera, Ant.crudum, Antimonium tart., Apocynum cannabinium, **ARANEA**., Arbutus andrachne, Arg.nit., Ars alb., Asterius, Aurum mur natronatum, *Bacillinum*, Baryta carb., *Benzoic acid*, Berb. vulg., *Bryonia*, Calc.carb., *Calc.iod.*, Cannabis sat, Carbo.sulph., Carbo.veg., Carbo an, Caulophyllum, **CAUSTICUM**, Chamomilla, **CONIUM**., Dulcamara., Graphites, Helleborus, Hepar sulph., Hyoscyamus, *Kali.sulph.*, Kalmia latifolia, *Lachesis, Lapis albus*, Ledum pal, Lilium tigrinum, Lithium carb, *Lycopodium*., Lycopus virginicus, Mag Phos, Mancinella, Mang.acet **MEDORRHINUM**, Mephities, Merc.cor, Merc. dulcis, Merc. iod. flavus, Merc. iod. ruber,

Merc. sulph, Murex, Mygale lasiodora, Myrica, **NAT.SULPH.**, *Natrum mur*, Natrum nitricum, **NIT. AC.**, Nitri spiritus dulcis, Ocimum can, Oleum santali, Oophorinum, Operculina turpethum, Origanum, Ostrya virginica, Oxydendron, Palladium, Pareira brava, Passiflora incar, Penthorum, Petroselinum, Phosphorus, Physalis, Piper methysticum, Pituitrin, Platina, Plumbum Met, **PULSATILLA**, **PYROGEN,** **RADIUM BROMIDE.**, Raphanus, Rhamnus cali., Rhodium, Rhododenron, Rhus tox, Rhus aromatica, Rhus glabra, Ruta grav., Sabal ser., Sabina., Sanguinaria nit, Sanicula, *Sarsap*, Scrophularia, Secal., Selen., **SEPIA,** Serum Anguillar, Sinnab., Solanum Lycopers, Spiranthes, **STAPHYSAG.,** Stellaria media, Sticta pulmonalis, Stigmata maydis, Stillingia, Stramo, Strontia, Strophanthus hisp, Strychnia, Sulfonal, Sulphur iod., Sumbul, Tannic ac., Tarantula hisp., Taxus baccata, Tellurium, Terebinth, Teucrium marum varum, Theridion, Thiosinaminum, Thlaspi bursa pastoris, **THUJA**, Thymol, **THYROIDINUM**, Torula cerevisiae, Tribulus terrestris, Triosteum perfoliatum, Tuberculinum, Turnera, Tussilago petasites, Uranium Nitricum, **URTICA URENS**, Ustilago maydis, Uva ursi, Vaccininum, **VARIOLINUM;** Veratrum album, Veratrum Vir, Viburnum Op, Viola Tricolor, Viscum Album, **X-Ray,** Yucca filamentosa, Zincum Met, Zingiber,

LEADING ANTI-SYPHILITIC MEDICINES:

Anthracinum, Arg nit., Arg.met., Ars. bromatum, Ars. metallicum, Ars.alb., Ars.iod., Artemisia vulgaris, Aurum.mur.nat., Asafoetida., Aurm.iod., **AURUM MET**., Aurum.brom., Badiaga, Baptisia, Calc.ars., *Calc.fl.*, Calc.iod.; Calc.s., Calendula, *Cannabis sat*, Cantharides, Carbo.an., Carbo.veg., Carbo.an., **CARCINOSIN., CINAB**., *Clematis.*, Conium., Corallium.rub., **FLUORIC ACID**., Guaiacum, *Hep.sulph.*, Hydrastis, **HYDROPHOBINUM**, Iodum., Kali.ars., **KALI.BICH.**, Kali.carb., **KALI.IOD**., Kali.mur., Kali.sulph., Kalmia., **KREOSOTE**., Lach., Ledum pal., Lycopodium, Manganum aceticum, Merc. iod flavus, *Merc.bin.iod.*, *Merc.bromatus.*, *Merc.cor.*, *Merc.cyan.*, *Merc.dulcis*, *Merc.iod.fl.*, *Merc.iod.rub.*, *Merc.proto iod.*, **MERC.SOL.**, **MEZEREUM**., Morphinum, Muriatic acid, Myristica seibifera, **NITRIC ACID**, Ornithogalum, Osmium., Paeonia, Petroleum., *Phos*, Phos.ac., Physostigma, **PHYTOLACCA**, Pyrogen, Ratanhia, Rhus Ven, Sabadilla, Sarsaparilla, Silicea, Solanum nigram, Spartium scoparium, **STELLARIA**., Stillingia, Sulphur, Sulphuric acid, Sulphurosum acidum, **SYPHILINUM**., Syzigium jambo, **TARANTULA CUB**, Thaspium aureum, Trifolium pratese, Trombidium, Tuberculinum.

LEADING ANTI-TUBERCULAR MEDICINES:

Acalypha ind., *Acet.ac.*, Agaricus muscarius, Ailanthus glandulosa, Allium cepa, Allium sat., Ammonium carbonicum, Ammon causticum, Antim tart., Arg nit., *Arnica mont.*, **ARS. IOD., BACILLINUM,** Baptisia, Baryta carb, *Belladonna*, Bromium, Bufo, Cactus grandiflorus, **CALC.CARB**., **CALC.IOD**., *Calc.phos.*, *Calc.sulph.*, *Carbo.an.*, Carbo.veg., *Carcinosin,* Chin.ars., **CHINA**, Cistus can, Conium mac., Crotalus horridus, Dros., Dulc., Elaps., Ferr.ars., Ferr.i., *Ferr.phos.*, Galium.ap., *Hamamelis vir.*, Helleborus, Hep. sulph, **HYDRAS.,** Hydrophobinum, Iberis, Ignatia, **IOD**., *Ipecac, Kali.c.*, Kali.chl., Kali.iod., Kali.nit., Kali.p., Kali.s., Lac.def., Lach., Lachnanth., Laurocer., Leptandra, Lyco., Mangifera indica, Merc cyanatus, Merc dulcis, Merc iod. flavus, Merc sol, **MILLEFOLIUM**, Muriatic acid, Naja tripudians, Natrum salicyclicum, Natrum nitricum, *Nit.ac.,* Oleum jec., Oxalicum acidum, Phelland., **PHOS. ACID**., **PHOS**., Pilocarpus, Plumbum met., Polygon.av., Psorinum, Sabina, Sang. Can., Santoninum,

Scrophularia nodosa, Secale Cor, Sempervivum tectorum, Senecio.aureus, Seneg., Sepia, **SILICEA**., Sinapis nigra, Skookum chuck, Solidago virga, Spigelia, Spong. tosta, Stann. Met., Strontia, *Sulphur*, Sulphuric acid, Taraxacum, Tarent. cub., Taxus Buccata, **TEREBINTH**, Theridion, **THLASPI BURSA PASTORIS**, Thyroidinum, Tilia europa, Titanum, **TRILLIUM PENDULUM**, Tri nitro toluene, **TUBERCULINUM**, Urea, Urtica urens, Verbascum, Vinca minor.

LEADING TRI-MIASMATICS:

Arg.Nit., Calcarea.Carb., Carcinosin, Causticum, Hydrophobinum (Lyssin), Hep.sulph., Lycopodium., Merc sol, Nitric acid., Phosphorus, Stellaria media, Sulphur, Tuberculinum.